Recent Research in Psychology

Bettina Hannover

Evaluation of Performance

A Judgmental Approach

Springer-Verlag
New York Berlin Heidelberg
London Paris Tokyo

Bettina Hannover
Institut für Psychologie
Technische Universität Berlin
1000 Berlin 10
West Germany

With 4 Figures.

Library of Congress Cataloging-in-Publication Data
Hannover, Bettina
  Evaluation of performance.
  (Recent research in psychology)
  Bibliography: p.
  1. Self-evaluation. 2. Performance. 3. Self-respect.
I. Title. II. Series.
BF697.H36   1988   155.2   88-11453

Camera-ready text prepared the author.
Printed and bound by Edwards Brothers, Inc., Ann Arbor, Michigan.
Printed in the United States of America.

9 8 7 6 5 4 3 2 1

ISBN 0-387-96768-0 Springer-Verlag New York Berlin Heidelberg
ISBN 3-540-96768-0 Springer-Verlag Berlin Heidelberg New York

*I am deeply grateful to J. Richard Eiser who
has read the manuscript several times
and has given me helpful suggestions
and criticisms. His support and inspiration
are appreciated more than I can say.*

Contents

Chapter 1

Self-evaluations of own performances as judgments: the internal standard

In achievement-related contexts, self-produced outcomes lead to self-evaluative reactions and to emotional experiences (Jucknat, 1938; Atkinson, 1957; Weiner, 1974, 1980; Heckhausen, 1977). Self-evaluations can basically be thought of as judgments, in that they involve the comparison of a perceptual input to some criterion. Classic research on the judgment of physical stimuli (e.g. Guilford, 1954) distinguishes between the internal or subjective representation of a set of stimuli (perceptual continuum) and the modality in terms of which the internal representation is expressed when a judgment is given (response continuum). This gives rise to the question of how the response continuum is 'anchored', that is, how different categories on the response scale come to be treated as equivalent to different stimulus values.

One view is that the perceptual continuum is fixed to the response scale at the mean stimulus (Helson, 1947). Another is that the extreme categories of the scale are anchored to the extremes of the response continuum or 'perspective' (Volkmann, 1951; Upshaw, 1962, 1969a, 1969b).

In research on self-evaluation, it is widely assumed that people set themselves certain performance standards and react to their own behavior in accordance with these self-imposed demands. Thus, self-evaluations result from the comparison of a perceived performance outcome with an internal standard (Atkinson, 1957; Bandura, 1974, 1977; Heckhausen, 1978, 1980; Kanfer, 1970, 1975; Kanfer & Hagerman, 1981; Kuhl, 1978, 1983a). Implicitly, it has been assumed that stimulus continuum (different levels of performance) and response scale are anchored at a single point, i.e. the self-imposed standard. Self-approving reactions occur if performance exceeds a standard, and self-criticism will follow if performance falls short of the standard. Little is known however, about how people acquire the standards that they use. As predicted by Bandura (1971) it has been shown that self-reinforce-ment-systems are transmitted by modeling, (Karoly & Kanfer, 1974; Bandura & Kupers, 1964; Bandura & Whalen, 1966; Bandura, Grusec & Menlove, 1967). Self-satisfaction or self-critical reactions are to a large extent determined by the models with whom a person compares him- or herself. The standard has always been treated as a factor that is internal to the individual. It has been assumed that people show a consistent and constant tendency to either use rather high or rather low self-rewarding standards (Atkinson, 1957; Kuhl, 1978). As a result, there has been no attempt to predict self-evaluative reactions, given a certain performance outcome, because the standard was considered as a parameter that could not be further specified. In addition, little attention has been paid to the question of how far a performance outcome has to exceed or fall short of the standard for self-approving or self-critical reactions to occur. It is to these issues that the present research addresses itself.

Bandura and Cervone (1983) have shown that both goal (standard) and feedback concerning performance outcome have to be experimentally induced in order for a positive covariation between self-dissatisfaction and subsequent intensification of effort to occur. Subjects had to perform a strenuous activity and were given either goals and performance feedback, goals alone, feedback alone or none of these. Self-dissatisfaction led to motivation enhancement only when both factors were present. These results can be interpreted as follows: people set them-selves different goals and may have different internal representations of the same performance outcome. If goals and feedback are not experimentally induced, "the mediating mechanisms are likely to operate variably depending on what partial information is available and on subjective provision of the missing comparative factor" (Bandura & Cervone, 1983, p. 1019). This may show that, in the absence of explicit goals or feedback, subjects may rely on different kinds of information in order to

define their standard and evaluate their own performance. As a result, no systematic covariation between
self-evaluation and motivation enhancement could be
shown. Indeed, 70 % of the subjects in the feedback-
alone-condition reported in a postexperiment
questionnaire that they had set performance standards on
their own. The expected differences in performance
enhancement could be shown if subjects were categorized
according to these self-set goals. Thus, self-evaluative
reactions and their motivational effects were dependent
on self-generated internal standards if only feedback was
given.

"...in the condition providing only feedback, knowledge of
a 24% gain in performance carried no absolute value. It
represented a commendable accomplishment if judged
against subjectively modest aspirations but a failure if
evaluated against subjectively invoked high standards.
Subjects' reports of their self-set goals reveal that many
of them either set no goals for themselves ...or aimed for
the same level of performance gain... For subjects in this
condition, a 24% gain constituted positive or success
feedback. The more pleased subjects were with sustaining
this level of improvement, the more effortfully they
behaved. In contrast, a 24% gain when one is aiming for
a 40% increment constitutes negative or failure feedback.
Discontent with the prospect of similar failure in the
future spurred subjects to greater effort. Inverted
meaning of the performance feedback thus produces
inverse relations between self-evaluation and performance
motivation" (p. 1026).

In our opinion, subjects' internal representations of
outcomes and subjects' individual standards are dependent

on the range of contextual informations made available in an experimental situation. Situational aspects that influence standard-height and outcome representation should be emphasized in order to predict self-evaluative reactions. Therefore, it is useful to assume that an internal continuum of performance outcomes and an external response continuum are not anchored at the self-imposed standard but rather at their extreme stimuli. People end-anchor the extremes of a given response modality with the extreme performance outcomes in order to evaluate own performances.

According to Upshaw's (1969a) theory of variable perspectives, central tendency and unit of judgments can be predicted if such a reference scale between stimulus perspective on the perceptual level and a certain response modality is known. Upshaw derives the central tendency of a judgment on a certain stimulus from the mean between the anchor stimuli, i.e. the two most extreme stimuli that form the boundaries of the perceptual perspective.

Perceptual perspectives in achievement-related contexts

In applying Upshaw's approach to self-evaluations of performances, the standard corresponds to the origin of the perceptual continuum and the unit to be used for judging deviations from the standard corresponds to the distance between the anchor stimuli. We are proposing that people use comparison stimuli that are available in a certain achievement situation to constitute a perspective on the basis of which evaluations of self-produced outcomes are formed. A perceptual continuum to be used for self-evaluations may consist of

- prior self-produced performance results;
- task-inherent properties, such as probability of success, by which a range of possible task difficulties is determined;
- performances of social comparison persons.

Prior self-produced performance results

The first source of stimulus-information has been dealt with in research on level of aspiration (Frank, 1935). It has been shown that (depending on previous performance results) people set themselves aspiration levels which in turn determine their judgments and affective reactions to performance outcomes (Jucknat, 1938; Lewin, Dembo, Festinger & Sears, 1944). Level of aspiration has been traditionally conceptualized as an aspect of the situation.

Each task has a positive valence for success and a
negative valence for failure. The more difficult the task,
the more positive the valence for success becomes, and
vice versa (Escalona, 1940; Festinger, 1942). Valences for
success and failure are then multiplied by the subjective
probability of success and failure, respectively. The
resulting valence, i.e. task choice or choice of aspiration
level, is equivalent to the product of success valence and
probability minus the product of failure valence and
probability (Lewin et al., 1944).

Task-inherent properties

Context information in the shape of task difficulty is
typically given in studies on achievement motivation.
Atkinson (1957) combined probability of success and
'incentive' in a stable mathematical function. In addition,
he introduced a person variable into the expectancy x
value model. Specifically, a motive to approach success
versus a motive to avoid failure was added as a
weighting factor to predict resulting motivational
tendencies. Achievement behavior is the result of an
emotional conflict between the tendencies to approach
success and to avoid failure. Looked at in this way
Atkinson's risk-taking model describes a system of self-
evaluation (cf. Heckhausen, 1977, 1980). Specifically, the
motives 'approaching success' versus 'avoidance of

failure' correspond to an emotional disposition to feel pride versus shame about success or failure. The incentive of success or failure is a self-evaluative emotion, the intensity of which is determined by task-difficulty. Specifically, the more difficult a task has been, the more intense is the positive affect following success. Preferred task difficulty and predominant achievement motive (Atkinson, 1957) have also been explained in attributional terms (Weiner & Kukla, 1970; Weiner, 1974). Specifically, the motives 'approaching success' versus 'avoidance of failure' correspond to different attributional styles in the case of success or failure feedback. Given success feedback, internal attributions occur if 'approaching success' is the predominant motive and external attributions are made if avoidance of failure predominates. However, with respect to failure feedback, differences mainly appear on the stability dimension. Specifically, attributions to unstable factors occur if approaching success is predominant. The opposite holds true if avoidance of failure predominates (cf. Frieze & Weiner, 1971; Kukla, 1972; Meyer, 1973). These results support the interpretation of achievement motives as self-reinforcement systems. Success orientation leads to the choice of intermediate task-difficulties as these allow for internal attributions in the case of success. Accordingly, avoidance of failure leads to the choice of either extremely easy tasks, so that success becomes very likely or extremely difficult tasks where an internal attribution for failure would seem rather inappropriate.

The intensity of emotional consequences is dependent on the difficulty of the task on which a person either succeeds or fails. By providing subjects with information about task difficulty a range of comparative stimuli is made available. If task difficulty is defined in terms of probabilities of success, a task can be ranked on a difficulty scale ranging from $p=0$ to $p=1$. The intensity of emotional consequences can be predicted if a self-evaluation scale is end-anchored to such a continuum of task difficulties: the closer the task difficulty is to the upper anchor ($p=0$), the more positive the resulting affect will be in the case of success. For failure, the nearer the task difficulty is to the upper anchor, the less negative the affect will be.

Performances of social comparison persons

Festinger's (1954) theory of social comparison processes is not particularly concerned with self-evaluations. Rather, following Festinger, social comparison processes enable one to find out about one's abilities and so to work out one's possibilities for action. As a result, empirical research on social comparison processes has been concerned with the question of which comparison persons are selected but has almost never looked at _effects_ of comparison processes. However, one of the theory's origins is the theory of reference group behavior (Merton & Rossi, 1949; Hyman, 1942). This is explicitly concerned with self-evaluations as consequences of the comparison of own performances to standards induced by the reference group. In addition, recent research has addressed itself to effects of social comparisons (cf. Halisch & Heckhausen, 1977; Brown & Inouye, 1978; Toda, Shinotsuka, McClintock & Stech, 1978; Seta, 1982; Harkins & Jackson, 1985), including self-evaluative affects (Masters, Carlson & Rahe, 1985).

So far, we have discussed different kinds of contextual information, in particular, previous own performance outcomes, task-inherent criteria and social comparison informations.

From the very same performance outcome, totally different self-evaluative reactions may result depending on the range of comparative stimuli that a person takes into account. The more positive the stimulus which forms the upper anchor of the internal continuum, the more negative self-evaluations on a certain performance outcome will be, assuming that the response modality is held constant. The opposite holds true for the lower anchor. The wider the distance between the anchors, the wider the unit by which deviations of a certain outcome from the standard are estimated (cf. Upshaw, 1969a).

Hence, changes in self-evaluative judgments can be expected from manipulations of the range of available contextual stimuli. However, it remains unclear whether changes in self-evaluation reflect changes in the internal representation of the performance outcome. It might be said that they simply correspond to changes in the way people define the verbal equivalents of a certain perceived performance result.

Scale effects versus changed stimulus-perception

Originally, in perspective theory the 'content of attitude' was distinguished from the 'judgmental attitude' or 'scale' (Ostrom & Upshaw, 1968). The same 'perceptual' stimulus (content of attitude) can be expressed in different categories of a given response modality depending on which attitude content a person associates with the extreme stimuli of a certain response scale (judgmental attitude or scale), i.e. changes in judgments may either reflect changes in stimulus-perception or changes in the reference scale. Ostrom (1970) conducted a study to operationalize the two conceptually different variables. Subjects learned of a person who had been found guilty of making a bomb threat in a hospital. They had to indicate the prison sentence they found appropriate (attitude content) and they had to rate themselves in terms of leniency–sternness (judgmental attitude or scale). Subjects were either committed to the content of their attitude or to the judgment: they had to write essays justifying content or judgmental attitude, respectively. Subsequently, different perspectives were induced. Specifically, different legal definitons of the presiding judge's discretion in sentencing were disclosed. As expected, subjects who had been committed to their attitude content changed their judgmental attitude according to the sentence range manipulation and those who had been committed to their judgment changed the content of their attitude. Only changes in attitude content were interpreted as changes of attitudinal position.

Related research was conducted by Upshaw (1978). In one experiment, Upshaw manipulated the self–proclaimed leniency–sternness of a judge along with the sentence he imposed. In a second experiment, he only varied the sentence and measured leniency–rating and sentencing as dependent variables. Changes in judgments would be interpreted as scale effects if they were to be observed only on those scales to which a manipulation directly pertained. Effects would have to be shown on both dependent measures for a change in attitudinal position to be assumed. Results supported the scale interpretation since effects only occured on scales that were directly manipulated. Hence, both content of attitude-ratings and judgmental attitude-ratings were interpreted as congeneric judgments, i.e. as reflections of the same unchanged attitudinal position. Changes occured because of changes in the response modality.

New criteria for distinguishing between attitude and response scale effects are introduced with the concept of congeneric scales (Upshaw, 1978; Upshaw & Ostrom, 1984). Congeneric scales are measures of the same property, which may differ in origin, unit or reliability but not in their factorial composition. If and only if changes in judgment occur on several congeneric scales, i.e. particularly on scales to which no perspective manipulation directly pertains, changes in judgment reflect changes in attitudinal position.

"An operation that anchors one congeneric scale to the stimulus continuum may have no effect on the anchoring of other scales. Hence, when the response range of one scale is extended by anchoring while the range of another remains intact, the expected result is assimilation to the remote anchor on the expanded scale, accompanied by no change on the other. (...) If the manipulation of extremity on one scale were found to affect respondent judgments on the other, this result would suggest that something more than the anchoring of two response scales had occured as a function of the manipulation. An obvious possibility would be that the manipulation had induced differences in respondent positions on the stimulus (attitude) continuum" (Upshaw, 1978, p. 330f).

There are important differences between the earlier and later versions of perspective theory with regard to the presumed causal links between judgmental and attitudinal effects. Specifically, in the earlier version (Ostrom & Upshaw, 1968; Ostrom, 1970) it was assumed that the sentence recommendation determines judgments on one's own leniency–sternness but not vice versa. Whereas the sentence recommendation reflects an attitudinal position, judgments only refer to scale effects. In the later version (Upshaw, 1978; Upshaw & Ostrom, 1984), the attitudinal position is a latent variable which determines both sentence recommendation and judgment.

Causal structures between stimulus–perception, judgments, and mood

In experiments to be reported in Chapter II, the latent variable is the internal representation of a self–produced performance outcome. Self–evaluations and mood are expected to covary with changes in how this outcome is perceived. That is to say, subjects are expected to give different judgments and to show mood changes with respect to own performances depending on manipulations of the range of available contextual stimuli. In considering whether these changes reflect changes in stimulus representation, we are assuming that the internal representation of a self-produced performance outcome has an immediate emotional effect. These "outcome-dependent affects" (Weiner, 1985) can be located (in simple terms) on a unidimensional scale from "good to bad" or from "sad to happy". They occur very quickly and are unescapably (Zajonc, 1980). However, in our opinion they are nevertheless the product of an individual learning process; spontaneous emotions are unconditioned or conditioned affective reactions (Leventhal, 1980). More precisely, we assume that people may represent a given outcome differently depending on a previous learning process and, as a result, are more or less likely to experience immediate positive or negative affects. Zajonc (1980) and Weiner (1985) differentiate between evaluatively positive and negative outcomes. However, they do not explain how people may experience an event as negative or positive in relation to some standard. People may experience the very same performance outcome as a success or a failure (as long as no such feedback is given by the researcher; cf. Bandura & Cervone, 1983). Weiner (1985) specifies that a certain intensity of the spontaneous affect is a necessary prerequisite for the occurrence of more diversified and prolonged emotions (which he calls "attribution-dependent"). However, he does not discuss the factors on which the negativity or positivity of a spontaneous outcome evaluation may depend.

Nonetheless, we will use Weiner's distinction between spontaneous and mediated affects. In our opinion, spontaneous affective reactions are dependent on the range of comparative stimuli a person takes into account. More precisely, the internal representation and the spontaneous affects associated with a certain outcome are dependent on the range of internally represented comparative outcomes. Therefore, immediate affective reactions are conditioned emotions (Leventhal, 1980, 1984) in as far as they are the result of a process of learning always to consider certain kinds of contextual information (for instance extremely positive information). Judgments, in particular self-evaluations, correspond to the <u>communication</u> of outcome-perception or of the internal affective state, respectively (Leventhal, 1980, 1984), and may produce affects in turn.

This view has the following implications for the interrelationships between stimulus representation, judgments, and mood.
Changes in judgment can either be due to a change in the internal representation of a performance result or can be due to a change in the way a person defines the verbal equivalent of a certain outcome. Changes in mood,

on the other hand, can be unequivocally interpreted as dependent on changes in the perception of the outcome. If mood worsens it can readily be assumed that the outcome is internally represented as more negative and vice versa.

Nevertheless, two different conceptualizations on the interrelatedness between self-evaluations and mood can be advocated.

- Mood and self-evaluations are congeneric scales (Upshaw, 1978), i.e. both self-evaluation and mood are response modalities into which the subjective representation of a certain performance outcome is linearly transformed. Self-evaluations and mood are multiple indicators of the latent variable 'internal representation of a self-produced outcome'.

- There are direct and mediated effects of the internal representation of a performance result on mood. Specifically, depending on the range of comparison stimuli considered, emotional effects result which may be suppressed by self-evaluations that exert an influence on mood in turn. Hence, in retrospect the stimulus may be perceived in accordance with mood.

The following empirical criteria are used to distinguish between scale effects and changes in the perception of the outcome. It is important to note that, in the following, the terms 'sufficient' and 'necessary' are not used in their logical sense and not used to set up a conceptual definition but only to fix an empirical criterion.

Changes in self-evaluative judgments are neither sufficient nor necessary for the assumption of a difference in the internal representation of performance outcome. Changes in mood, on the other hand, are sufficient and even necessary conditions of such an assumption (particularly if possible suppression effects of self-evaluative judgments are taken into account).

When we come to consider our experiments, it should be noted that no manipulation of mood was included. Specifically, perspective manipulations refer to self-evaluations but not to mood. In addition, even if a mood-related manipulation were to be given, we would not expect changes in mood ratings to occur as simple effects of scale anchoring. More specifically, we would argue that mood as an internal state determines mood ratings but not vice versa (even though Upshaw's, 1978, formulation might suggest otherwise). Whereas self-evaluations are built up according to the context to which a certain stimulus is judged, mood ratings first of all refer to a given internal state the communication of

which is not so dependent on the situation. We assume that people use a reference scale that consists of
- a stimulus continuum of internal states which is constricted by the extreme emotional states a person has experienced and
- a response continuum of verbal expressions to communicate mood.

If the response scale is held constant it is fair to assume that a change in mood scores indicates a real change in an internal affective state as long as no extreme emotional states are induced which might possibly change the internal continuum of previously experienced emotions. That is to say, an internal perspective of mood states is used with relatively high consistency and stability. In addition, mood is the most direct operationalization of the internal representation of an outcome that one can think of. Naturally occuring events coincide with spontaneous affects (Weiner, 1985) or lead to unconditioned or conditioned emotional reactions (Leventhal, 1980, 1984) which are not cognitively mediated. It is likely that the internal representation of the outcome will be different, i.e. the emotional experience will be dissimilar, if a manipulation of contextual stimuli to be used to judge own performances leads to changes in mood scores. To apply the original distinction from perspective theory (Ostrom & Upshaw,

1968), mood corresponds to "attitude content" whereas self-evaluations correspond to the "judgmental attitude" or "scale".

Why are changes in self-evaluations neither necessary nor sufficient criteria for changed stimulus-perception? They are not sufficient because perspective manipulations in our experiments directly pertain to self-evaluative judgments (cf. Upshaw, 1978). They are unnecessary because they are judgments that not only serve a communicative but also an emotion-regulatory function (v. Cranach, Kalbermatten, Indermühle & Gugler, 1980; Lantermann, 1982, 1983; Kuhl, 1983b; Brandstädter, 1985; Dörner, 1985). Self-produced outcomes lead to spontaneous affective reactions (Weiner, 1985; Metalsky, Halberstadt & Abramson, 1987). Presumably, not only the outcome but the judgment as such exerts an emotional effect. That is to say, stimulus-perception has direct and mediated influences on affective state. Specifically, negative effects of failure on mood may be prevented by positively distorted judgments of own performance outcomes. Thus, in order to suppress negative effects on mood, a negative internal representation of an outcome may not be reflected in corresponding self-evaluations. By denying or minimizing perceived failure, negative affect is prevented. As a result, in retrospect the outcome may be perceived in accordance with mood.

The existence of such a structure can be assumed if the following pattern were to be found in empirical data: a negative performance result (as compared to a range of available contextual outcomes) has a negative effect on mood which is suppressed by a positively distorted self-evaluation.

To summarize, in our experiments two different causal structures are interpreted as indications of changed stimulus representation. A change in perspective that may lead to a more negative stimulus- perception should either result in corresponding changes in both self-evaluations and mood or it should result in positively distorted judgments which in turn suppress a negative effect on mood.

Choice of perspectives

Ordinarily, individuals are exposed to a variety of possible standards against which they may judge a particular stimulus. It has been shown in several empirical studies that people judge stimuli only with respect to those contextual standards they consider as relevant (Brown, 1953; Parducci, Knobel & Thomas, 1976;

Manis & Paskewitz, 1984a, 1984b; Manis, Paskewitz & Cotler, 1986). In other words, contrary to Helson's (1947) assumption, not all the available contextual informations are automatically reflected in the adaptation level, or standard used when judging a given stimulus. Applied to perspective theory, a perceptual perspective is not necessarily constricted by the two most extreme stimuli.

Perspective theory is unspecific as to what stimuli people take into account to form a perceptual perspective.

"In assessing the present status of perspective theory, we are led to the conclusion that its most critical deficiency is a lack of principles by which to account for the range of content positions that a person considers in forming, changing, and judging an attitudinal position. Surely, information from external sources is a major determinant of this variable within the theory. However, there are certainly processes within the person that interact with external information to produce the effect" (Upshaw & Ostrom, 1984; p. 38).

We maintain that, depending on certain situational or motivational demands, people either use the total range of available comparative stimuli, or only parts of the perceptual continuum, to build a judgmental perspective.

People may use peripheral stimulus information or correlated cues to subdivide the total range of perceptual stimuli into different "sub-perspectives". Hence, they may use only parts of the total range of stimuli to judge a certain stimulus. Kahneman and Miller (1986) discuss a similar assumption as a "local norm" and Higgins and Lurie (1983) refer to a similar phenomenon as a "subjective norm". A study conducted by Manis, Paskewitz and Cotler (1986) provides empirical support for the proposition that people may evaluate a certain stimulus with reference to different contextual stimuli in the same judgment situation. They found a local intraclass contrast effect that was due to subjects' using a correlated cue to judge a particular stimulus only with respect to contextual stimuli of its own class.

We expect people to use only parts of the range of contextual stimuli to define their perspective if hot cognitions as opposed to cold cognitions (Zajonc, 1980) are at issue. Judgments of self-produced performance outcomes are hot cognitions in as far as they have emotional effects. A desire to evaluate own performances accurately can be differentiated from a tendency to upgrade own performances (cf. Singer, 1966 and Goethals & Darley, 1977: "evaluation versus validation of the self"; Thornton & Arrowood, 1966 and Latané, 1966: "self-evaluation versus self-enhancement"; Austin, 1977: "objective evaluation versus protection of self-esteem"; Brickman & Bulman, 1977: "adaptive versus hedonic forces"). In broad terms, it can be said that the use of the whole range of available comparative stimuli leads to accurate self-evaluation. In a desire to positively judge own performances, on the other hand, contextual stimuli at the upper end of a perceptual continuum should be neglected.

Specifically, we expect a tendency for subjects to narrow down the range of their perspective in situations in which self-esteem is threatened. This is because a perspective with lowered origin heightens the probability of reaching a positive evaluation of self-produced outcomes. Positive self-evaluations may be functional to protect self-esteem or to prevent negative mood effects.

Aspects of response language

The notion that people anchor a certain response scale to a perceptual continuum at the most extreme stimuli they can think of has also been challenged by the work of Eiser and his associates. Interactions between judges' attitudes and evaluative aspects of the response language on polarization could be shown if subjects had to judge stimuli on two or more scales which differed only in their evaluative meanings (Eiser & Mower White, 1974, 1975; Eiser & Osmon, 1978; Eiser & van der Pligt, 1982). Following the distinction introduced by Peabody (1967), descriptive, i.e. denotative, and evaluative, i.e.

connotative, aspects of response language can be differentiated. In the studies mentioned above, the denotative description of a stimulus continuum was held constant and at the same time its connotative aspects were varied. The following pattern emerged: On scales with a connotatively positive pro-end, judges with a pro-attitude polarized more than judges with anti-attitude, and vice versa. Perspective theory (Upshaw, 1969a) would account for polarization as an effect of scale unit. More specifically, the larger the distance between the anchors of the perceptual perspective, the less polarization should occur. In its original formulation (Upshaw, 1962) perspective theory cannot explain results showing that more polarized judgments occur for extreme pro-judges than for neutral subjects and more polarized judgments for neutral subjects than for anti-judges (e.g. Zavalloni & Cook, 1965). Eiser (1973) ascribes these results to an influence of the evaluative meaning of the response language: in the studies in which asymmetrical polarization for pro- and anti judges was found, subjects were confronted with response scales of which pro-anchors were connotatively positive. Thus, for anti-judges evaluative consistency could best be maintained by giving less polarized judgments thereby avoiding giving a connotatively extremely positive rating to items with which they disagreed or an extremely negative rating to items with which they agreed.

Eiser and van der Pligt (1982) tried to test the distinct predictions of accentuation and perspective theory. They used an experimental design that was modeled on Upshaw's (1962) experiment, but provided subjects with several response modalities which were different with respect to value connotations. An interaction between judges' attitudes toward the issue and the range of presented items was to be expected according to perspective theory. Specifically, Upshaw (1962) predicted effects of own attitudes for "out-of-range" judges (those whose own position lay beyond the range of items presented) but not for more moderate "in-range" judges. Since a clear differentiation between in- and out-of-range judges seems difficult, Eiser and van der Pligt conceived of an interaction between width of presented item-range and judges' attitudes as support for perspective theory. The wider the item-range, the fewer subjects will be "out-of-range". Hence, differences in polarization as a function of judges' attitudes should be larger, when the range of items is narrow. However, no such interaction was found, which was at odds with perspective theory. On the other hand, they found an interaction between value connotations of response language and judges' attitudes, as predicted by accentuation theory. Perspective theory can account for judgmental changes arising from manipulation of response

language. However, Upshaw would dispute that the
response language as such may have a direct influence on
perspective. On the other hand, it seems inappropriate to
assume that subjects in Eiser and van der Pligt's study
changed their perspectives each time a differently labeled
response scale was presented. Eiser and van der Pligt are
led to the conclusion that the response modalities are
less arbitrarily anchored to a certain perceptual
continuum than Upshaw maintains.

"...it is assumed that subjects may approach a judgment
task with prior notions concerning the appropriateness of
a particular response scale for judgments of a particular
dimension, or ranges of positions along a dimension"
(p.229).

Eiser and van der Pligt interpret their results as
indication that people match the response language to an
appropriate range of stimuli. More concretely, response
scales with an evaluatively positive pro-anchor are
appropriate to judge (attitudinal) items ranging from
extremly anti up to moderately pro and response scales
of which the anti-anchor is positive seem appropriate to
judge items ranging from moderately anti up to extremly
pro. Such a view seems compatible with perspective
theory

"if one moves from the original definition of perspective
as the total range of positions a person can think of to
a definition based on a conception of the range of
positions it seems appropriate to compare in terms of a

particular judgmental language" (Eiser & van der Pligt, 1982, p.238).

This interpretation is challenged by Upshaw and Ostrom (1984). They dispute that denotations and connotations of a set of stimuli can be manipulated independently. Hence, the different scales with which subjects were provided in Eiser's studies would not meet the requirements of congeneric scales. In their opinion, connotatively different scales pertain to different content sets. Eiser (1986) counterargues

"that, while A+ and P+ scales differ in denotation, they still can be assumed to denote regions of the same content dimension. There may be differences in the means and standard deviations of ratings on the different scales, but the scales may still intercorrelate. If this is so, there is no reason why the different scales should not be regarded as 'congeneric' " (p. 168).

With respect to our line of reasoning, the controversy is to be interpreted in the following way. We have maintained that people tend to neglect stimuli at the upper end of a perceptual continuum under threat to self-esteem. In the light of Eiser's results, we suppose that threat can additionally lead to a 'reluctance' to use a certain response modality. Specifically, threat may intensify the tendency to contrast a judgment away from an evaluatively negative anchor of the response scale if one's own position were to be placed near that anchor. In our experiments, subjects were provided with failure feedback on their own performances. Hence, judgments of own performances were to be given near the lower anchor if the induced perspectives were normatively used. Contextual stimuli at the upper end of a perceptual continuum are expected to be neglected if self-esteem is threatened. In addition, subjects should contrast their judgments away from the lower anchor if that anchor of the response modality is evaluatively negative. A main effect would be expected for threat and additionally an interactive effect from threat and connotation if threat and connotation of response language were manipulated independently: people should neglect positive perceptual stimuli, thus giving more positive judgments of their own performances when under threat. Moreover, judgments should be additionally contrasted from the lower response scale anchor under threat if that anchor is evaluatively negative. Threatened subjects should use the scales differently as opposed to unthreatened subjects if more than one response scale is offered.

In our opinion, response scales which differ in their evaluative meaning can be conceived of as congeneric scales. They are used differently, however, because a self-related negative judgment as such has negative effects on mood. In Upshaw's (1978) opinion, the interactive effects between attitudes and connotation of response language in Eiser's studies are effects of social desirability or response scale stretching.

"Presumably, a socially desirable definition of responses in the vicinity of one's own extreme scale position encourages the use of responses in that region because it results in the presentation of one's own position as socially desirable. Such an effect amounts to a functional expansion of the response range for those subjects compared to others whose positions fall elsewhere on the scale" (p. 330).

For self-evaluative judgments of own performances, such an interpretation is rendered superfluous: to contrast judgments from an evaluatively negative anchor is functional to maintain or protect self-esteem and to prevent negative mood.

These hypotheses have to remain speculative, since, for reasons of sample size, threat and connotation of response language were not manipulated independently in our experiments. Rather, in Experiment I, a response scale was provided of which the lower anchor was evaluatively negative whereas in Experiment II the response modality was evaluatively neutral. Thus, more positive judgments should appear in both experiments if threat leads to the neglect of stimuli at the upper end of a perceptual continuum. Correspondingly, no effects of the threat manipulation should appear in the second experiment if threat leads solely to a refusal to use evaluatively negative response modalities.

Threat to self-esteem

'Threat' is a variable that has been conceptualized many different ways. Threat may lead to better stimulus discrimination and at the same time to lowered sensitivity in the processing of peripheral stimuli (Erdelyi & Appelbaum, 1973) or to distortions in judgments (Upmeyer, 1976). Upmeyer (1981) illustrates such a view in reinterpreting Asch's study of the effects of group pressure on judgment (Asch, 1951).

"We have argued that judgmental distortion operates on and is limited to the response process, whereas perceptual distortion as a result of social pressure occurs during the process of internal representation of stimuli; however, contrary to Asch, we feel that this perceptual process can hardly be described as distortion due to the fact that persons subjected to social pressure improve their perceptual performance... (...) When others are of a different opinion... with respect to some reality..., the self feels threatened, resulting in a closer inspection and an improved internal representation of all aspects of that reality...; if reality in this situation is ambiguous... and the social sanctions are perceived to be strong..., the self will most likely yield to the others... " (Upmeyer, 1981, p.281).

Other authors have discussed different ways of dealing with threatening information as person-specific cognitive styles (Gordon, 1957; Miller, 1980, 1987).

Threat to self-esteem has been operationalized as receipt of information that is negatively discrepant from a person's self-concept (Johnson, 1966; Hamilton, 1969; Wyer & Frey, 1983; Frey, Stahlberg & Fries, 1986). It could be shown quite consistently that people consider those dimensions on which negative self-related informations are received as less important (Lewecki, 1983; Frey & Stahlberg, 1987) or as less "self-definitional" (Tesser & Campbell, 1980).

In the context of our experiments, we are particularly interested in effects of threat to self-esteem on the search for contextual stimuli to be used for evaluating self-produced performance outcomes. There is empirical support from experimental studies (Hakmiller, 1966; Wilson & Benner, 1971; Friend & Gilbert, 1973; Sanders, 1981) and from applied research (Taylor, Wood & Lichtman, 1983; Wood, Taylor & Lichtman, 1985; Molleman, Pruyn & van Knippenberg, 1986) that upward comparisons are functional in situations of self-esteem threat. Wills (1981) argues that downward comparisons lead to increased subjective well-being if people experience negative affects. In our opinion, downward comparison can be interpreted as an indication that people extend the range of comparative stimuli, i.e. their perceptual perspective, at the lower anchor and neglect information at the upper anchor. Applied to achievement-related contexts, as a result, they may upgrade judgment of own performance. We assume that failure perception is threatening to self-esteem if and only if the negative outcome is considered as strongly self-definitional; in other words, if the outcome is on a dimension that is critical to one's self-concept. This should lead subjects to judge their own performances more positively.

In our experiments, half of the subjects were threatened in their self-esteem. All subjects were given failure feedback since they were outperformed to either large or moderate extents by an experimental confederate. Threat to self-esteem, however, was induced by the experimenter's focussing on the subject's inferiority and the confederate's superiority, respectively. This operationalization of threat is similar to the one used by Wilson and Benner (1971). Here, subjects were given fictitious moderate feedback about their own results in a test of leadership abilities. The dependent measure was a comparison choice of another group member's test-score. Subjects were either led to believe that the result of the comparison would be publicly announced or that it would only be made available to the subject ("public/private manipulation"). Results confirmed the expectation that, in the public comparison situation, subjects avoided comparing themselves with the highest ranking person because they were concerned with the possibility of an unfavorable comparison-result which would threaten self-esteem. In contrast, in the private situation subjects' primary motive was to maximize information, resulting in their choosing the highest ranking person as a comparison point.

The threat manipulation used in our experiments is similar to the public/private manipulation in Wilson and Benner's (1971) study. Specifically, in the threat conditions, the fact that the confederate outperformed the subject is mentioned by the experimenter as opposed to the no-threat conditions in which the subject's inferiority goes unnoticed.

We expected subjects to distort judgments of own performances positively if acknowledgement of a negative performance outcome would threaten self-esteem. It was hypothesized that this would be the case if the confederate's superiority was emphasized by the experimenter. Hence, we expected that subjects would not use the most extreme available stimuli to build a perspective under threat to self-esteem. Rather, stimuli at the upper end of a perceptual continuum should be neglected. As a result, own performances could be judged more positively, given that the origin of the perspective is lowered. It was anticipated that threatened subjects would exclusively use the perspective of which the upper anchor was relatively low if more than one perspective was made available.

With respect to the causal structure between stimulus-perception, self-evaluation, and mood, the following differences were expected depending on the threat manipulation. Ordinarily, outcome- perception should be simultaneously reflected in both self-evaluative judgments and mood. Self-evaluative and mood-scales are multiple indicators of the latent variable 'internal representation of the outcome'. This is to say that, without threat, both self-evaluations and mood should be more negative in the context of a perspective with a high origin (or central tendency) as compared to a perspective with a low origin. Under threat to self-esteem, however, the effects of performance perception were expected to be mediated by self-evaluations. Specifically, we anticipated positively distorted judgments under threat which in turn would have positive effects on mood. As a result, neither threat as such nor the perception of a negative performance outcome under threat should have negative effects on mood.

Actual self-evaluations and global self-esteem

The self-concept is the sum of self-related judgments, i.e. the ascription of traits and person characteristics to oneself (cf. Stroebe, 1977). Whereas these self-related judgments are value-neutral, self-evaluations correspond to the affective components of these judgments. The weighted sum of these affective self-evaluations is the self-esteem of a person (Frey & Benning, 1983). These definitions are in accordance with the assumption of a summation rule in information processing (Fishbein & Hunter, 1964). In our opinion, there are several reasons for such a conceptualization to be criticized. First of all, there is no empirical support for the proposition that self-esteem is the sum of self-evaluations. In addition, with a summation rule it is implied that self-evaluations are compensatory and that the direct contribution of each single self-evaluation to the global self-esteem is simply its value at the time it is formed. That is to say that actual self-evaluations are independent of self-esteem.

There are several objections to these assumptions. Specifically, it can be doubted whether the effect of an extremely negative and an extremely positive self-evaluation on self-esteem is equivalent to the contribution of two evaluatively moderate self-evaluations. Moreover, it has been shown that self-esteem becomes more stable over the life span (Mummendey & Sturm, 1978, 1980). It appears, the more frequent self-evaluations already occurred or the larger the range over which previous self-evalutions are distributed, the less influential an actual self-evaluation is. In addition, the processing of actual self-related information seems to be dependent on a person's self-esteem, i.e. on previous self-evaluations (Canon, 1964; Korman, 1968; Skolnick, 1971; Dutton, 1972; Mettee & Aronson, 1974; Brewer & Campbell, 1976; Shrauger & Terbovic, 1976; Smedley & Bayton, 1978; Bornewasser, 1985).

Hence, we maintain that the self-concept of a person is not sufficiently described by the algebraic sum of all previous self-evaluations. Rather, it seems that range and frequency distribution of previous self-evaluations have to be taken into account. Whereas actual self-evaluations are sufficiently explained by the range principle (Volkmann, 1951; Upshaw, 1962, 1969a), frequency effects (Parducci, 1963, 1965) have to be considered additionally with respect to the self-concept.

We hypothesize that self-evaluations of own performances are cumulatively entered into a so-called "life perspective" which can be conceived of as the estimate of one's own achievement capability (in the following referred to as a person's achievement-related "self-concept"). The life perspective can be modeled as a bipolar scale. The endpoints of this scale are defined by the extremes of previous self-evaluations, between which a frequency distribution of self-evaluations emerges over time. Specifically, a rectangular distribution results if negative and positive self-evaluations are entered with the same frequency into the life perspective. Accordingly, a negatively or positively skewed distribution results from more frequent positive or more frequent negative events respectively. In our model, the subjective representation or the "self-concept" of one's own achievement capability depends on the distribution on the life perspective. Self-esteem corresponds to the modal stimulus of the frequency distribution. The reasons for these assumptions are as follows.

Parducci (1984) has suggested that reactions of happiness and unhappiness depend upon the distribution of a person's previous happy and unhappy experiences. Applying the range-frequency principle (Parducci, 1965) in a relational theory of happiness, Parducci (1984) expects a positively skewed distribution of contextual events to lead to more negative evaluations of an actual stimulus, and vice versa. The general level of all value judgments corresponds to the happiness of a person. Happiness is determined by a person's subjective neutral point which in turn is dependent on the range and the distribution, in particular the skewing of the distribution, of contextual events. The neutral point is the modal value judgment. From the fact that the skew of a distribution can be roughly estimated from the difference between mean and modal value divided by the dispersion of values (Bortz, 1985) it can be inferred that a positively skewed context of events leads to more negative judgments as compared to a negatively skewed context of events. This holds true even if the mean value of events in the positively skewed distribution is above the one of the negatively skewed context of events (cf. Parducci, 1984).

In our model, the distribution on the life perspective exerts the same influence on actual judgments. However, this is for another reason: the distribution represents the part of one's self-concept relating to one's own achievement capability. The modal stimulus on the life perspective (the person's self-esteem) may be used as a "third variable" or a "correspondence cue" under uncertainty (Upmeyer, 1981): If a person is unsure as to whether a certain stimulus, in our case a self-produced performance outcome, is representative of response category R_1 or response category R_2, he or she may take into account a third variable category which is psychologically related but different from the stimulus variable. The person will be more likely to respond R_1 if the third variable is more correspondent with stimulus S_1 than with stimulus S_2 and vice versa (cf. Upmeyer, 1981, p. 274). Accordingly, actual self-evaluations tend to be more negative if the distribution on a person's life perspective is positively skewed, and vice versa. To put it into other words, the distribution on the life perspective functions as an expectancy of stimulus frequency.

"The concept of expectation can also be viewed as a special case of the correspondence principle in operation, the third variable in this case consisting of the frequency of response occurrence. The similarity between the concepts is heightened by the fact that both are based on the observer's past experience" (Upmeyer, 1981, p. 275).

Parducci starts out from the idea that actual value judgments are constituted relative to range and frequencies of other events in the context, i.e. frequency information has to be processed in separate contexts of events. In our model, all self-evaluations are entered into a single life perspective. We maintain that actual judgments are fairly adequately explained by the range principle. As we see it, the processing of frequency information in different event- contexts is much too complex a cognitive process to be plausibly assumed (cf. Haubensak, 1981). Over time, a frequency distribution of self-evaluations develops on the life perspective. The self-esteem as the modal stimulus can function as a "third variable" or a "correspondence cue". That is to say, under uncertainty actual self-evaluations are distorted in the direction of the highest density of the frequency distribution on the life perspective. A cognitively much more simplistic process is presupposed with the assumption that people use frequency information from their own self-concept, given that the self-concept is relatively stable over time. The assumption that the general self-esteem retroacts on actual self-evaluations is consistent with empirical results on the interrelatedness between general self-esteem and information processing. If self-esteem is significantly lowered, negative informations about the self are sought (Dutton, 1972) and self-serving informations are depreciated (Shrauger & Lund, 1975). It seems, self-oriented informations are processed holistically in the light of the global self-esteem (cf. Asch, 1946).

Etiology of unipolar depression
In applying our theoretical model to explain unipolar depressions the following restrictions have to borne in mind. Psychological theories on depression are disproportionately cognitive in emphasis. In general, cognitive processes have been considered as causally relevant to the emergence of unipolar depression.

Consequently, environmental factors, namely real life-conditions, have been disregarded as possible antecendents of depression (cf. Coyne & Gotlib, 1983). Empirical research has almost exclusively been concentrated on cognitive variables, like attributions, contingency expectations, and probablility estimates. Very rarely have researchers considered the question of whether certain cognitive features are really depression-specific. Although causal relationships between cognitions and depression have been claimed, these relationships typically have not been empirically tested (Coyne, 1982). Therefore, Brewin (1985) argues, certain cognitive features may as well be consequences of depressive mood states, or may just describe more or less efficient styles of coping with depressive affects (cf. also Harvey, 1981).

Within the predominant cognitive interpretation of depression it is explicitly or implicitly assumed that cognitions are causally antecedent to emotions. Such an unidirectional conceptualization of the relationship between emotion and cognition runs counter to the recent work of several authors who emphazise the effects of emotional processes on cognitions (i.e. Bower, 1981; Kuhl, 1983c). Following Weiner (1985), we have distinguished spontaneous from mediated affects. The former can be conceived of as unconditioned or conditioned emotions (Leventhal, 1980); they may appear as reactions to naturally occurring life-events. They are prerequisites for the emergence of 'cold cognitions' (Zajonc, 1980), for instance attributions, and therewith also prerequisites for mediated specific emotions (Metalsky et al., 1987). However, the application of our model is restricted to achievement situations. Accordingly, only experiences of success or failure are taken into account as possible spontaneous affects. It is important to note that we do not at all conceive of a negative self-concept of own achievement capability or of failure experiences in achievement situations as necessary or even as sufficient causal conditions for the emergence of unipolar depressions. With our model we merely want to emphasize that

- affects are not just epiphenomena of cognitive processes or just their consequences. Affects occur immediately and, in addition, they exert a cumulative effect over time: in the long run they function as an expectation;
- an interdependence of emotional and cognitive processes has to be assumed.

Conceptually, we are talking about depression. In our empirical studies, however, we induce a situationally negative mood. It is by no means maintained that the latter is identical with the former. Rather, we assume that negative affects exert a cumulative effect over time which is mediated by their influence on an expectancy of the person (life perspective). To be more precise, negative situational affects are dissimilar from depression but cumulative effects of negative mood may possibly produce a depression-resembling emotional state. Intervening variables, by means of which spontaneous negative affects may lead to a vicious cycle of increasingly negative emotions, are not especially dealt with here. However, this should be no means taken to imply that they can be safely neglected.

Psychological theories describe the symptoms of depression as follows (cf. Ellis, 1962; Beck, 1967, 1976; Seligman, 1975). Depressives show
- a lowered motivation to produce volitional behavior;
- cognitive deficits (that in detail are conceptualized differently by different authors);
- emotional deficits, namely a generalized dysphoric mood together with lowered self-esteem, feelings of worthlessness, and self-blame.

How do our theoretical assumptions relate to the etiology of unipolar depression? Development of depression is a process that is extended over time. Specifically, it is expected that a positively skewed distribution emerges on the life perspective which corresponds to a lowered self-esteem if negative self-evaluations occur more frequently than positive ones over a prolonged period of time. Depressives can be characterized by an extremly positively skewed distribution on their life perspectives.

For a positively skewed distribution to develop, actual self-evaluations have to be consistently negative. Inherent to our theoretical approach as described so far, this should occur if persons tend to take into consideration extremely positive or only moderately negative contextual information to provide the upper or lower anchors of a perceptual perspective, respectively.

"Many of the people who seek psychotherapy... experience a great deal of personal distress stemming from excessively high standards of self- evaluation often supported by unfavorable comparisons with models noted for their extraordinary achievements. (...) In its more extreme forms, a harsh system of self-reinforcement gives rise to depressive reactions, chronic discouragement, feelings of worthlessness, and lack of purposefulness. (...) As Loeb, Beck, Diggory and Tuthill (1967) have shown, depressed adults evaluate their performances as significantly poorer than do nondepressed subjects, even though their actual achievements are the same" (Bandura, 1971, p.31).

Empirical evidence that depressives have heightened aspiration is inconsistent (Frese & Schöfthaler-Rühl, 1976). In our opinion, this is due to the overlooked possibility that depressives may tend to generate a negative internal representation of performance outcomes. Both the tendency to use raised standards and to distort stimulus-perception negatively, may lead to depressive reactions.

Our assumption that depressives use perceptual perspectives with raised origins is supported by results from life event research (Katschnig, 1980; Filipp, 1981). Experiences of extremely negative events may, if they are successfully coped with, serve as negative perspective anchors. This in turn may lead to more positive evaluations of other events (cf. Sledge, Boydstun & Rabe, 1980).

We have discussed some evidence that nondepressed people react to threat with intensified self-serving judgments. Such a pattern could be interpreted as the adaptation of perceptual perspectives to situational demands (cf. Hakmiller, 1966; Sanders, 1981; Wood et al., 1985; Molleman et al., 1986). It seems that people with significantly lowered self-esteem do not react to situational threat with such self-protective judgmental distortions (Dutton, 1972; Shrauger & Lund, 1975). The self-esteem of depressives is definitely lowered (Laxer, 1964; Nadich, Gargan & Michael, 1975; Pagel & Becker, 1987). It appears that depressives do not adapt perceptual perspectives to situational demands (Tabachnik, Crocker & Alloy, 1983; Tesser, 1984). Rather, they show less positively biased judgments than nondepressives

(Lewinsohn, Mischel, Chaplain & Barton, 1980; Abramson & Alloy, 1981; Coyne, 1982; Coyne & Gotlib, 1983; Wollert, Heinrich, Wood & Werner, 1983; Taylor & Brown, 1986). Hence, self-serving biases can be conceived of as protective factors against depression (Klein, Fencil-Morse & Seligman, 1976; Alloy & Abramson, 1979, 1982; Abramson, Alloy, & Rosoff, 1981; Alloy, Abramson & Viscusi, 1981; Metalsky, Abramson, Seligman, Semmel & Peterson, 1982; Raps, Peterson, Reinhard, Abramson & Seligman, 1982; Martin, Abramson & Alloy, 1984; Vázquez, 1987; Tennen & Herzberger, 1987).

Reviewing literature on evaluative tendencies of nondepressed, mildly, and severely depressed people, Ruehlman, West, and Pasahow (1985) come to the conclusion that, with respect to judgments of contingency, causal attributions, expectancy estimates and self-schemata

"nondepressed people tend to exhibit positivistic evaluative responses, whereas mildly depressed persons tend to display unbiased (neither positivistic nor negativistic) evaluative response patterns. The available evidence is suggestive of negativistic evaluative tendencies in severely depressed individuals, with this bias being most clearly manifested in the area of self-schemata /self-reference" (p.46).

These results are consistent with our hypotheses: with increasing number of previous negative self-evaluations the skew of the frequency distribution becomes more and more positive. Self-esteem is lowered, thus additionally retroacting negatively on actual self-evaluations. The positive skew of the frequency distribution increases exponentially.

Our assumptions, concerning the predominant use of perceptual perspectives with raised origins, remain speculative. Nevertheless, predictions concerning further development can be specified if a positively skewed distribution on the life perspective is assumed.

Parducci (1984) does not consider the possibility that the happiness of a person, i.e. his or her general level of value judgments, may in turn affect expectations on the frequency distribution of certain events in a given context (since he is not especially interested in processes that are extended over time). With our model, the following temporal development of the distribution on the life perspective can be expected. If the distribution is asymmetrical, the entering of further stimuli is more likely to increase the degree of skew than to make the distribution more normalized. More concretely, a positively skewed distribution on the life perspective heightens the probability of the occurrence of negative actual self- evaluations which in turn intensify the positive skewness. Under uncertainty, actual judgments are distorted in the direction of the highest density of the distribution (cf. Upmeyer, 1981). This can explain how depressive tendencies emerge over time and tend to become more intense (Ruehlman, West & Pasahow, 1985). Depression can be described as a self–maintaining system of negative self– evaluations (Ellis, 1962; Beck, 1976).

Given a positively skewed distribution, the probabilty of the occurrence of negative events in the future is relatively or absolutely overestimated. This is because the distribution on the life perspective operates like an expectancy of stimulus frequency. Probabilities for future events are estimated by projecting the frequency distribution onto a response modality. That part of the distribution with the highest density is reflected in more response categories (Parducci, 1965). Thus, depressives anticipate more negative events (Alloy & Ahrens, 1987). As motivated behavior is guided by the anticipation of positive consequences (Bandura, 1978; Heckhausen, 1977; Kanfer, 1975; Weiner, 1974), this leads to a lowered motivation and activity level. This in turn not only results in less frequent positive self–reinforcement but also in fewer external reinforcements (Lewinsohn, 1974).

So far, we have maintained that depressives use perspectives with raised origins, and this leads to more frequent actual negative self–evaluations and negative mood affects (Masters et al., 1985). Over time, a positively skewed distribution on the life perspective emerges. The decreased self-esteem is used as a correspondence cue under uncertainty. A self-maintaining system of negative self-evaluations is established. Prolonged negative mood originates

- from actual negative self-evaluations that coincide with negative affects and
- from the frequency distribution. Specifically, negative events are anticipated and because of the lowered self-esteem actual self-evaluations are additionally negatively distorted.

Roughly, Weiner's (1985) distinction between spontaneous and distinct emotions can be applied to these different sources of affects. Weiner distinguishes between spontaneous, outcome-dependent and distinct, attribution-dependent emotions. Outcome-dependent, attribution-independent emotions simply reflect goal attainment or nonattainment. Following outcome appraisal, different causal ascriptions will be sought, and each of these will be related to a set of distinct emotions like pride, hopelessness, surprise, shame, guilt and so on. In our opinion, actual self-evaluations correspond to outcome-dependent emotions and effects of the frequency distribution correspond to distinct emotions.

In terms of perspective theory, actual self-evaluations may be simple "scale" effects. Specifically, people may use a reference scale that is made available in a certain situation. However, self-evaluations as such are expected to produce corresponding affects. Moreover, self-evaluations are entered into the life perspective, thus contributing to the global self-esteem which in turn retroacts on actual self-evaluations. This notion is supported by empirical results showing effects of experimentally manipulated self-presentations on the global self-esteem (Gergen & Taylor, 1969; Morse & Gergen, 1970; Ickes, Wicklund & Ferris, 1973).

Thus, self-evaluations, even though they may simply reflect an anchoring process, have immediate and (by means of their contribution to self-esteem) prolonged affective consequences. Moreover, the outcome may in retrospect be perceived as more negative if negative affects occur as a result of negative self-evaluations.

Weiner (1985) is particularly interested in attribution-dependent emotions. However, he emphasizes that outcome-dependent emotions (with a certain intensity) are necessary prerequisites for causal ascriptions to be sought. A study conducted by Metalsky, Halberstadt and Abramson (1987) shows that outcome-dependent affects are a prerequisite for the appearance of attribution-dependent emotions. This study tested a "cognitive diathesis-stress theory of depression" (Abramson, Alloy & Metalsky, 1986; Abramson, Metalsky & Alloy, 1986), essentially a refinement of the reformulated helplessness theory of depression (Abramson, Seligman & Teasdale, 1978). The tendency to attribute negative events to internal, stable, and global causes is conceived of as a diathesis for depressive reactions, whereas negative life events are conceived of as stressors. This new model attempts to clear up ambiguities in the original (Seligman, 1975) and reformulated helplessness theory (Abramson et al., 1978) concerning the causal structure and the temporal aspects of any causal sequence (Cochran & Hammen, 1985) between variables concerning the person (perception of control or attributional style, respectively) and the occurrence of certain events (uncontrollable or negative events, respectively) with respect to their effects on mood. In addition, the reformulated helplessness theory was unclear on the question of whether both attributional style and negative events or only one of these components were necessary for depressive reactions to appear.

The diathesis-stress model (Abramson, Alloy & Metalsky, 1986) specifies a causal mediation of the effects of negative events on mood by attributional ascriptions.

Metalsky et al.'s (1987) results are important within the present context since they support the view that negative immediate outcome-dependent affects are a necessary prerequisite for the emergence of prolonged negative affects.

"...the logic of the reformulation suggests that in the presence of positive life events or in the absence of negative life events, people exhibiting the hypothesized attributional diathesis should be <u>no more likely</u> (emphasis added) to develop depressive reactions accompanied by lowered self-esteem than should people not displaying the hypothesized attributional diathesis" (p. 386f).

Metalsky et al. measured attributional styles (diathesis) of students and their results on a class midterm exam, categorized as failure (stress) or success corresponding to a difference score between goal and result. The following data pattern was expected. For students who had experienced failure, general attributional styles were anticipated to be predictive of particular attributions for the low midterm grade and of subsequent depressive mood responses. Additionally, these students' attributional styles should not have a direct effect in predicting subsequent depressive mood beyond that of the particular attribution for the midterm grade. The effects of the attributional diathesis on mood-responses to failure should be mediated by students' particular causal attributions for the low grades. Results were only partially consistent with Metalsky et al.'s hypotheses.

Immediate depressive mood reactions were solely predicted by the outcome of the midterm exam. Unexpectedly, the interaction-term between attributional style and midterm outcome did not contribute significantly to the prediction of immediate depressive mood responses. On the other hand, consistent with the diathesis-stress theory, prolonged affects as measured two days later were solely predicted by this interaction term. More concretely, independent of attributional style negative mood emerged immediately from a negative outcome. Two days after receipt of the grade, however, only students with global and stable attributional style for negative events showed enduring negative affects as opposed to students with specific and instable attributional style who had completely recovered from their spontaneous depressive reaction.

Metalsky et al.'s (1987) results are consistent with our theoretical assumptions. If and only if the midterm exam was considered a failure, immediate and prolonged depressive mood reactions occurred. At odds with Metalsky et al.'s hypotheses, the perception of failure was a sufficient condition for negative mood to occur, i.e. a depressive attributional style was not necessary.

To use Weiner's (1985) terms, the immediate mood reactions are equivalent to outcome-dependent emotions and prolonged emotions correspond to attribution-dependent distinct emotions. Neither Weiner (1985) nor Metalsky et al. (1987) considered factors that influence immediate outcome-dependent affects. If spontaneous emotions reflect goal attainment or nonattainment it can be said that, depending on standard height or on person-specific tendencies to internally represent outcomes as positive or negative, corresponding attribution-independent emotions should occur with different frequency.

As Bandura & Cervone (1983) have shown, people generate goals and feedback on themselves. Only if clear-cut feedback of success or failure is given can one predict what the resulting outcome-dependent emotion will be like. If no such feedback is available, people may generate different "subjective feedback" on the very same performance outcome.

In our model it is assumed that the internal representation of an outcome, i.e. the subjective feedback, is dependent on the range of comparative stimuli a person takes into account. In our opinion, factors influencing perspectives that are used to evaluate performance outcomes should be emphasized since they determine immediate affects which in turn are prerequisites for the appearance of distinct emotions.

Our model does not allow for an explanation of the use of different attributional ascriptions. However, with our theoretical approach special weight is given to the consideration that depressed people may first of all be characterized by a tendency to generate negative spontaneous feedback, i.e. to represent self-produced performance outcomes negatively.

To summarize, in our opinion actual self-evaluations which can be predicted by means of the range principle correspond to outcome-dependent affects; distinct emotions are dependent on the distribution of self-evaluations on the life perspective. Hence, people who consistently use perspectives with raised origins experience negative outcome-dependent affects more frequently and give more frequent negative judgments of self-produced performances. As a result, distinct negative emotions occur more frequently as well.

With our model, the symptomatic deficits of depressives can be conceptualized as follows.
- Self-produced outcomes are consistently internally represented as negative because perceptual perspectives with heightened origin are used and, in addition, because the lowered self-esteem, as the modal stimulus on the life perspective, is used as a correspondence cue. As a result, negative mood as outcome-dependent

emotion is more likely to occur. Distinct emotions result from attributional processing of success and failure (Frieze & Weiner, 1971; Abramson, Alloy & Metalsky, 1986). In other words, distinct emotions emerge from the processing of spontaneous emotions. Actual self-evaluations that can be described by the range principle correspond to outcome-dependent emotions and distinct emotions are dependent on the frequency distribution on the life perspective. Specifically, it can be assumed that self-evaluations are entered into the life perspective only if performance outcomes are internally attributed. As a result, they influence self-esteem. This is in line with empirical results showing that outcomes have effects on self-esteem only if they are attributed to internal causes (Stipek, 1983; Weiner & Handel, 1985).

- The distribution on the life perspective functions like an expectancy of stimulus frequency. Negative self-evaluations are expected to occur more often than positive ones (Alloy & Ahrens, 1987). Achievement motivation has been described as a self-reinforcing system (Atkinson, 1957; Heckhausen, 1977). The anticipation of positive consequences motivates volitional activity (Bandura, 1971, 1978; Kanfer, 1975). These consequences can either consist of external reinforcement or of self-produced consequences of one's actions, i.e. self-approval or self-blame. If no self-satisfaction is expected, volitional activity decreases. As a result, not only self-produced (Smolen, 1978; Lobitz & Post, 1979) but also external positive reinforcement occurs less frequently (Lewinsohn, 1974; Goodhart, 1986).

- The cognitive deficit can be conceptualized as a lowered capability to adapt actual judgmental perspectives to situational demands. In more concrete terms, such a deficiency may be due to an incapacity to generate standards that are appropriate to specific situations.

Summary of hypotheses

Let us summarize our theoretical assumptions and the ways in which they will be tested.

- Judgments of performance outcomes and corresponding mood are predictable from the parameters of a perspective of which the anchors are the most extreme stimuli available. An interaction effect between order of induction and time of measurement is expected if subjects are provided with a wide perspective with high origin and a narrow perspective with lower origin at two measurement points, balancing the order of induction: judgments and mood should become more positive from time 1 to time 2 if the wide perspective is induced first, but more negative if the narrow perspective is induced first.

- Subjects should not use the whole range of available stimulus information if self-esteem is threatened. If subjects have more than one perspective available, they will tend to choose the perspective with the relatively lowest origin as this will enable greatest self-esteem protection. This should lead to a main effect for threat and a three-way interaction between threat, order of perspective-induction, and time of measurement. Specifically, judgments and mood are expected to be more positive under threat. For unthreatened subjects, judgments and mood should become more negative from time 1 to time 2 if perspectives are induced in the order 'narrow-wide' and become more positive to the same extent in the 'wide-narrow' order condition. On the other hand, for threatened subjects, judgments and mood should become more positive in the 'wide-narrow' condition but remain unchanged in the 'narrow-wide' condition.

- Self-evaluative judgments of own performances have effects on mood. Only if no self-esteem threat is present would mood be expected to be a congeneric scale onto which the internal representation of a self-produced outcome is linearly transformed in the same way as onto self- or other- oriented judgments. If self-esteem is threatened, however, positive distortions in judgments are expected which in turn improve mood, i.e. the internal representation of a stimulus is not simultaneously reflected onto different response modalities. Whereas for unthreatened subjects direct effects of the experimental manipulations on all dependent variables are expected, effects may be mediated for threatened subjects.

- Self-evaluations are not only dependent on the parameters of a situational perspective but also on judgments that occurred in the past. Specifically, the person who shows a positively skewed distribution on his or her life perspective is expected to judge stimuli as more negative. A skewed distribution develops over a prolonged period of time. Applied to a single experimental session in which judgments are measured at two separate occasions, a more positive skew at the second point of measurement as compared to the first is interpreted as indicative of such a mechanism. In addition, the more negative judgments actually are, the more positive the skew should be. Specifically, the higher the origin of the perspective which is used to judge a series of stimuli the more positive the skew of the distribution of judgments is expected to be.

Chapter 2

Experiment I

Method

Subjects

Subjects were 60 male adolescents between 12 and 24 years of age, who were recruited by newspaper advertisement. For participating in the two-hour experimental session they were paid 20 German marks. Subjects were run in single sessions (with an experimental confederate) and were randomly assigned to experimental conditions.

Stimulus materials

Videotapes of computer-game plays functioned as stimuli for a standard set of objects of judgment and as experimental manipulations of perspectives. The computer game involved guiding a little man through a maze, with more and more complex levels being reached as one progressed. Specifically, a videotape showing a play from the first level up to the 30th level served as "large perspective" and a tape from the first level up to the 18th level as "narrow perspective".

It was ensured that both tapes showed plays which were much better than those of the subjects. A standard set of outcomes consisted of videotapes of a total of twelve plays on one level each. The range of standard deviations obtained from pretest ratings of the difficulty of the standard set stimuli was 0.0 to 2.2. on an 11-point-scale.

Procedure

When subject and confederate arrived for the experiment, the experimenter explained the computer game. It was emphasized that the subject's and confederate's play would be videotaped and shown to them afterwards. Subject and confederate were each seated in front of a personal computer each. They both played for 20 minutes. Subsequently, they were told that only the videotape of the better of the two performances would be shown. For half of the subjects, it was emphasized by the experimenter that the videotape would show the confederate's play (self-esteem threat manipulation). One of the two perspective-videotapes was presented (induction of first perspective). Subsequently, the standard set of outcomes was shown to the subjects. Subjects had to rate each outcome and their own performance in terms of positivity. Subjects completed a depression inventory. Thereupon the experimenter pretended to show the performance of another, anonymous person. The videotape of the other perspective was shown (induction of second perspective). The order in which the perspectives were induced was balanced between subjects (wide-narrow versus narrow-wide). Again subjects had to rate the standard set outcomes and their own performance and to complete a depression inventory. Subjects were debriefed and paid.

Dependent measures

Standard set ratings and evaluations of own performance (self-evaluation) were measured on a visual analog scale. Specifically, subjects had to put magnets on a scale that was painted on a metal ledge of which the end-anchors were marked by a "smiling" and a "crying face", 190 cm apart.

Mood was measured with two parallel versions of a standardized depression inventory that is sensitive to situational mood swings (v. Zerssen, 1976).

Task performance was examined to rule out any differential performances between groups.

Results

Task performance data

A one-way ANOVA computed on performances showed significant differences between groups ($F_{(3,56)}=5.67$, p=.002). A Scheffé-test showed that the subjects in the self-esteem threat condition with the wide perspective induced at the first point of measurement performed significantly better than subjects in each of the other three groups and that the other groups did not differ significantly from each other.

Therefore it was impossible to perform any analyses of covariance in order to partial out the effects of performances on the dependent variables.

Effects of threat to self-esteem

Analyses of variance for repeated measures (2x2x2) were performed on all dependent variables testing for effects of self-esteem threat and order of perspective induction.

Results for the standard set ratings were as follows:

A significant main effect for the threat manipulation on mean standard set ratings (first moment of the distribution) was obtained $(F_{(1,56)}=12.65, p=.001)$. Threatened subjects gave more positive judgments than unthreatened subjects did.

No interactive effects between threat manipulation and the other factors were found. The three-way interaction between threat, order of perspective-induction, and time of measurement was not significant $(F_{(1,56)}=1.726, p=.191)$.

For each subject, standard deviations on ratings of all standard set stimuli (second moment of the distribution) were computed. Analysis of variance for repeated measures yielded no main effect for the threat manipulation ($F_{(1,56)}=1.88$, p=.17). Again, the three-way interaction was not significant ($F_{(1,56)}=.605$, n.s.).

For each subject, the degree of skew of standard set ratings (third moment of the distribution) was computed. Analysis of variance showed a significant main effect for the threat manipulation ($F_{(1,56)}=6.76$, p=.01). Overall, threatened subjects produced a more negative skewness than unthreatened subjects did.

For self-evaluations and mood, results were as follows: There was only a marginally significant effect of the threat manipulation for evaluation of own performance ($F_{(1,56)}=3.08$, p<.08) and no effect at all for mood ($F_{(1,56)}=1.99$, n.s.). Instead, for both variables a significant interaction between threat manipulation and order manipulation was found ($F_{(1,56)}=7.06$, p<.01 for self-evaluation; $F_{(1,56)}=4.3$, p=.04 for mood). Whereas the threatened subjects gave more positive self-evaluations and reported a better mood in the wide-narrow condition, the opposite was true for unthreatened subjects. An analysis of covariance with repeated measures on mood with the effect of self-evaluation partialled out yielded a marginally significant main effect for the threat manipulation ($F_{(1,56)}$=3.08, p=.08). As opposed to the marginally significant main effect on self-evaluation, mood was more negative in the threat condition. For both variables, the three-way interaction was not significant ($F_{(1,56)}$=.125, n.s. for self-evaluation; $F_{(1,56)}$=.082, n.s. for mood).

Effects of perspectives

For all dependent variables, analyses of variance for repeated measures showed a significant interaction effect for order of perspective-induction and time of measurement: whereas in the wide-narrow condition mean standard set ratings, self-evaluations, and mood were more positive at time 2, the opposite held true for the narrow-wide condition ($F_{(1,56)}$=22.85, p<.001 for mean standard set ratings; $F_{(1,56)}$=11.18, p=.001 for self-evaluation; $F_{(1,56)}$=5.71, p=.019 for mood). Dispersions of standard set ratings were smaller at time 2 in the narrow-wide condition but larger in the wide-narrow conditions ($F_{(1,56)}$=7.55, p=.008). Aggregated over all groups, a slightly negative skewness was found (Mean=-.136). There was no significant interaction between order of perspective-induction and time of measurement for skewness (F < 1). Instead, a significant main effect was found for skewness. The distribution was more positively skewed at the second point of measurement ($F_{(1,56)}$=19.57, p<.001).

Comparison between expected and observed values

If subjects used the induced perspectives for their judgments, perspective theory should allow for a deterministic prediction of absolute judgment values. The normative or expected parameters were computed by dividing the number of response categories (160) by the number of objects that constituted the particular experimental perspective (30 and 18 objects for wide and narrow perspective, respectively). The resulting quotient is the unit of the perspective. The unit was multiplied with the height of each standard set object. The mean expected standard set judgment is equivalent to the mean value of judgments on all single objects. Expected standard deviations are equivalent to the dispersion of the expected mean judgments on all objects.

To compute expected self-evaluations, mean performances per experimental group were multiplied with the theoretical unit that was computed by means of the above mentioned procedure.

For computation of expected mood scores, the same procedure was used. As high scores corresponded to bad mood (high depression) the scores were transformed by the following equation:

$y = -1$ (performance x unit) + number of response categories.

Difference scores between expected and observed values were computed for all dependent variables. The difference scores were divided by the dispersion of the observed values. Due to the small sample sizes, the resulting value is t-distributed.

To test for the equivalence between expected and observed standard deviations, the product of degrees of freedom and sample variance was divided by the expected population variance. The resulting Chi2-values were used for two-tailed testing.

All observed values were tested against the expected values of both perspectives (wide and narrow) at both points of measurement. It was speculated that the two induced perspectives were combined into a "compromise perspective" at the second point of measurement. Therefore, observed values at the second point of measurement were tested against the expected values of a perspective of which parameters were interpolated by averaging the parameters of the two induced perspectives.

Table 1. (cf. pp. 70 and 71) shows the results for the first point of measurement for the standard set rating.

Results showed that at the first point of measurement observed values could be predicted by the parameters of the induced perspective only in the "no threat, narrow—wide condition" (t=0.23[1], p=.50[2]). In all other conditions, the observed values were better explained by hypothetical perspectives that were narrower than the

---

[1] In all tables, t—values refer to the comparison between observed mean ratings and expected values. Expected values are the mean ratings which were to be anticipated if subjects had used the actually induced perspective. For instance, an observed mean rating at t1 in a narrow—wide-condition is compared with the mean value which were to be expected if subjects had used a perspective with a range of 18 game-levels (narrow perspective). Positive t—values indicate that the subjects judged more positively than would have been predicted, and vice versa.

[2] Because of an unspecific hypothesis (i.e. that observed values are not significantly different from expected values) the β-error could not be computed. Therefore, p's are indicated up to an α-level of 50% in all tables.

TABLE 1.
Comparison expected and observed values,
standard set rating t_1

N = 60	observed mean (SD)	used perspective[1]	expected mean (SD)	expected mean (SD) other perspect.
Condition				
n = 15 threat wide perspective[3]	85.7 (24.5)	$x_1 = 17.7$ $x_2 = 9.0$	50.7 (18.4) t=7.37 p<.01[2] chi^2=24.7 p<.10[4]	84.4 (30.7) t=0.16 p=.50[2] chi^2=8.9 p=.50[4]
n = 15 threat narrow perspective[5]	107.0 (39.2)	$x_1 = 14.2$ $x_2 = 11.3$	84.4 (30.7) t=2.85 p<.05[2] chi^2=22.9 p<.10[4]	50.7 (18.4) t=11.85 p<.01[2] chi^2=63.5 p<.01[4]
n = 15 no threat wide perspective[3]	64.4 (21.9)	$x_1 = 23.6$ $x_2 = 6.8$	50.7 (18.4) t=2.88 p<.05[2] chi^2=19.7 p=.50[4]	84.4 (30.7) t=2.53 p<.05[2] chi^2=7.1 p<.30[4]
n = 15 no threat narrow perspective[5]	86.3 (32.4)	$x_1 = 17.6$ $x_2 = 9.1$	84.4 (30.7) t=0.23 p=.50[2] chi^2=15.6 p=.50[4]	50.7 (18.4) t=7.48 p<.01[2] chi^2=43.7 p<.01[4]

Note.

 [1] x1=range   x2=unit

 [2] Comparison between observed and expected mean values
t emp for df=14; two-tailed test

t crit(14;50%) = 0.692   t crit(14;70%) = 1.076

t crit(14;80%) = 1.345   t crit(14;90%) = 1.761

t crit(14;95%) = 2.145   t crit(14;99%) = 2.977

 [3] range x1 = 30   unit x2 = 5.33

 [4] Comparison between observed and expected standard deviations
chi^2emp for df=14; two-tailed test

chi^2crit(14;50%) = 10.1653 and 17.117

chi^2crit(14;80%) =   7.7895 and 21.064

chi^2crit(14;90%) =   6.5706 and 23.685

chi^2crit(14;95%) =   5.6287 and 26.119

chi^2crit(14;99%) =   4.0746 and 31.319

 [5] range x1 = 18   unit x2 = 8.89

induced ones. In the condition "threat, narrow-wide", the observed values were explained by a hypothetical perspective that had a range of x=14.21[1]. Such a perspective is almost identical with a perspective that is restricted by the lowest object of the perspectives and the highest standard set object, respectively[2]. Possibly the standard set as such was used as a judgmental perspective. The positively distorted observed mean judgments coincided with greater dispersions with the exception of the "no-threat, wide-narrow condition".

Results for the second point of measurement for the standard set rating are shown in Table 2. (cf. pp. 74 and 75).

In the threat condition, observed values were best described by the narrow perspective (t=1.13, p<.30). Without threat, the hypothetical perspective which best described observed values was the compromise perspective

---

[1] The range of the induced perspective in this condition was x=18, i.e. the videotape showed a play from the first level up to the 18th level of the game (narrow perspective).

[2] The highest standard set object was a play on the 15th level of the game.

(t=0.14, p=.50 for wide−narrow condition; t=0.45, p=.50 for narrow−wide condition). Observed dispersions were some−what smaller than would have been predicted for the perspectives which explained the observed mean judgments.

Table 3. (cf. p. 76) shows the results for self−evaluations for the first point of measurement and Table 4. (cf. p. 77) for the second one.

Aside from the "threat, wide−narrow condition", observed values at the first point of measurement were best explained by the expected values of the induced perspective (t=−.96, p<.30 for "threat, narrow−wide condition"; t=−0.14, p=.50 for "no threat, wide−narrow condition"; t=−1.1, p<.30 for "no threat, narrow−wide condition"). Again with the exception of the "treat, wide−narrow condition", observed self−evaluations at the second point of measurement were best described by a compromise perspective (t=0.02, p=.50 for "threat, narrow−wide condition"; t=−1.35, p<.20 for "no threat, wide−narrow condition"; t=−1.2, p<.30 for "no threat, narrow−wide condition). As compared to the standard set ratings, self−evaluations were less positively distorted.

TABLE 2.
Comparison expected and observed values,
standard set rating t_2

N = 60	observed mean (SD)	used perspective[1]	expected mean (SD) other perspect.	expected mean (SD)	expected mean (SD) compromise perspect.
Condition					
n = 15 threat narrow perspective[3]	93.4 (23.8)	x_1=16.3 x_2= 9.9	84.4 (30.7) t=1.126 p<.30[2] chi[2]=8.4 p=.50[4]	50.7 (18.4) t=8.98 p<.01[2] chi[2]=23.5 p=.50[4]	63.3 (23.0) t=5.05 p<.01[2] chi[2]=15.0 p=.50[4]
n = 15 threat wide perspective[5]	82.4 (22.2)	x_1=18.5 x_2= 8.7	50.7 (18.4) t=6.67 p<.01[2] chi[2]=20.3 p=.50[4]	84.4 (30.7) t=0.26 p=.50[2] chi[2]=7.3 p<.20[4]	63.3 (23.0) t=3.21 p=.01[2] chi[2]=13.0 p=.50[2]
n = 15 no threat narrow perspective[3]	62.5 (20.6)	x_1=24.4 x_2= 6.6	84.4 (30.7) t=2.78 p<.05[2] chi[2]=6.3 p<.10[4]	50.7 (18.4) t=2.48 p<.05[2] chi[2]=17.5 p=.50[4]	63.3 (23.0) t=0.14 p=.50[2] chi[2]=11.2 p=.50[4]
n = 15 no threat wide perspective[5]	66.0 (21.9)	x_1=23.0 x_2= 7.0	50.7 (18.4) t=3.22 p<.01[2] chi[2]=19.4 p=.50[4]	84.4 (30.7) t=2.33 p<.05[2] chi[2]=7.2 p<.10[4]	63.3 (23.0) t=0.45 p=.50[2] chi[2]=12.7 p=.50[4]

Note.

[1] x1=range   x2=unit

[2] Comparison between expected and observed mean values
t emp for df=14; two-tailed test

t crit(14;50%) = 0.692   t crit(14;70%) = 1.076
t crit(14;80%) = 1.345   t crit(14;90%) = 1.761
t crit(14;95%) = 2.145   t crit(14;99%) = 2.977

[3] range x1 = 18   unit x2 = 8.89

[4] Comparison between observed and expected standard deviations
chi^2emp for df=14; two-tailed test

chi^2crit(14;50%) = 10.1653 and 17.117
chi^2crit(14;80%) = 7.7895 and 21.064
chi^2crit(14;90%) = 6.5706 and 23.685
chi^2crit(14;95%) = 5.6287 and 26.119
chi^2crit(14;99%) = 4.0746 and 31.319

[5] range x1 = 30   unit x2 = 5.33

TABLE 3.
Comparison expected and observed values,
self-evaluations t_1

N = 60	observed mean (SD)	used perspective[1]	expected mean (SD)	expected mean (SD) other perspect.
Condition				
n = 15 threat wide perspective[3]	76.4 (54.0)	$x_1 = 21.2$ $x_2 = 7.5$	54.0 (16.2) t=5.36 p<.01[2]	90.1 (26.9) t=1.97 p<.10[2]
n = 15 threat narrow perspective[4]	52.8 (28.3)	$x_1 = 19.8$ $x_2 = 8.1$	58.1 (21.5) t=-0.96 p<.30[2]	34.8 (12.9) t=5.4 p<.01[2]
n = 15 no threat wide perspective[3]	46.1 (31.0)	$x_1 = 30.3$ $x_2 = 5.3$	46.6 (15.3) t=-0.14 p=.50[2]	77.6 (25.4) t=-4.8 p<.01[2]
n = 15 no threat narrow perspective[4]	63.9 (32.7)	$x_1 = 19.5$ $x_2 = 8.2$	69.3 (19.3) t=-1.1 p<.30[2]	41.6 (11.6) t=7.42 p<.01[2]

---

[1] x_1=range x_2=unit

[2] Comparison between expected and observed mean values
t emp for df=14; two-tailed test
t crit(14;50%) = 0.692   t crit(14;70%) = 1.076
t crit(14;80%) = 1.345   t crit(14;90%) = 1.761
t crit(14;95%) = 2.145   t crit(14;99%) = 2.977

[3] range x_1 = 30   unit x_2 = 5.33

[4] range x_1 = 18   unit x_2 = 8.89

TABLE 4.
Comparison expected and observed values,
self-evaluations t_2

N = 60	observed mean (SD)	used per- spective[1]	expected mean (SD)	expected mean (SD) other perspect.	expected mean (SD) compromise perspect.
Condition					
n = 15 threat narrow per- spective[3]	94.2 (37.4)	x_1 =17.2 x_2 = 9.3	90.1 (26.9) t=0.59 p=.50[2]	54.0 (16.2) t=9.63 p<.01[2]	67.5 (20.2) t=5.1 p<.01[2]
n = 15 threat wide per- spective[4]	43.6 (27.2)	x_1 =24.0 x_2 = 6.7	34.8 (12.9) t=2.64 p<.05[2]	58.1 (21.5) t=2.64 p=.05[2]	43.6 (16.1) t=0.02 p=.50[2]
n = 15 no threat narrow per- spective[3]	51.6 (35.5)	x_1 =27.1 x_2 = 5.9	77.6 (25.4) t=-3.96 p<.01[2]	46.6 (15.3) t=1.27 p<.20[2]	58.2 (19.1) t=-1.35 p<.20[2]
n = 15 no threat wide per- spective[4]	47.5 (25.1)	x_1 =26.3 x_2 = 6.1	41.6 (11.6) t=1.97 p<.10[2]	69.3 (19.3) t=4.38 p<.01[2]	52.0 (14.5) t=-1.2 p<.30[2]

---

[1] x1=range   x2=unit

[2] Comparison between expected and observed mean values
t emp for df=14; two-tailed test
t crit(14;50%) = 0.692   t crit(14;70%) = 1.076
t crit(14;80%) = 1.345   t crit(14;90%) = 1.761
t crit(14;95%) = 2.145   t crit(14;99%) = 2.977

[3] range x1 = 18   unit x2 = 8.89

[4] range x1 = 30   unit x2 = 5.33

Observed mood scores were transformed into standard T-scores before they were tested against expected values.

In all experimental groups, observed values were definitely higher than the values of all hypothetical perspectives. It was hypothesized that subjects might have used only parts of the response scale. Judging own mood at the "upper anchor" of the depression inventory would have been equivalent to saying that one was in an extremely and clinically depressed state. Possibly subjects exclusively used the upper two thirds of the response scale, i.e. perhaps they end-anchored the stimulus continuum with a scale that consisted of the lower two parts of the response modality only. Expected values were computed for a reduced response scale range. Specifically, the original scale from 0 up to 56 points (the higher the score, the more intense depression is) was constricted to a range from 0 to 48.

Comparisons between observed and expected values again resulted in clearly lower observed than theoretical values except for the condition "no threat, narrow-wide". It was concluded that absolute values of mood scores could not be predicted with any of the hypothetical perspectives.

Causal structures

To clarify the causal structure between the experimentally manipulated and the dependent variables a multiple regression approach was used. All variables that precede a variable in a specified theoretical model were simultaneously entered as predictors into a multiple regression analysis. Independent variables were treated as exogenous variables in a path model. Due to the significant performance differences a complete model for the whole sample could not be computed. The prerequisite of exogenous variables to be uncorrelated was not met. Models for subgroups of threatened versus unthreatened subjects were specified. It is important to note that interpretations of the model for the threatened subpopulation are preliminary because effects of order manipulation and performance were confounded. Following Upshaw (1978), path-analytic models in an after-only design, i.e. after induction of the first perspective, were computed. The exogenous variable 'size of perspective' (wide versus narrow) was dummy-coded. Causal links between the variables of a specified causal model were estimated from the sample covariance matrix. Pearson product-moment correlation coefficients for the subpopulations of threatened and unthreatened subjects are provided in Table 5.

TABLE 5.

Intercorrelations for threatened subjects, Experiment I

	1.	2.	3.	4.
1. Perspective				
2. Performance	.55**			
3. Self-evaluation	.35	.43*		
4. Standard set rating	-.43*	-.27	.09	
5. Mood	-.06	-.16	-.41*	.23

Note. n=30.
*p<.05. **p<.01.

Intercorrelations for unthreatened subjects, Experiment I

	1.	2.	3.	4.
1. Perspective				
2. Performance	.18			
3. Self-evaluation	-.28	.36*		
4. Standard set rating	-.36*	-.12	.39*	
5. Mood	.47**	-.19	-.39*	-.22

Note. n=30
*p<.05. **p<.01.

Using the order in which the different measures were obtained to specify a "causal structure" the following models resulted.

FIGURE 1.

Threat conditions

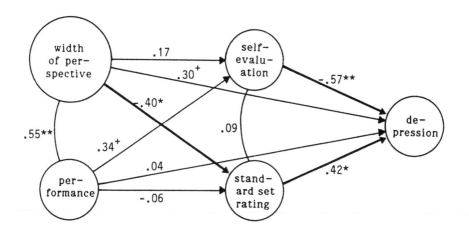

Note.
Only qualified interpretation is possible; cf. text.
n=30.
+p<.10. *p<.05. **p<.01.
t-values were as follows.
beta=.34, t=1.68, p<.10
beta=.30, t=1.35, p<.10
beta=-.40, t=-1.91, p<.05
beta=-.57, t=-2.86, p<.01
beta=.42, t=2.16, p<.05
For all other coefficients t<1.0, n.s.

FIGURE 2.

No threat conditions

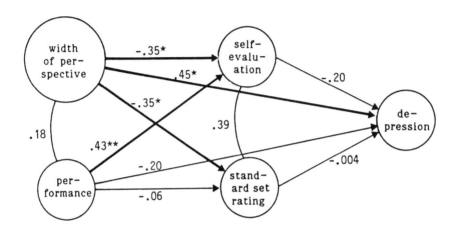

Note.
n=30.
*p<.05. **p<.01.
beta(perspective, self-evaluation)=-.35, t=-2.09, p<.05
beta=.45, t=2.42, p<.05
beta=.43, t=2.52, p<.01
beta(perspective, standard set rating)=-.35, t=-1.92
For all other coefficients t<1.0, n.s.

If the standard set rating was included as an additional predictor the path coefficients were as follows.

FIGURE 3.

Threat conditions. Standard set rating as an additional predictor

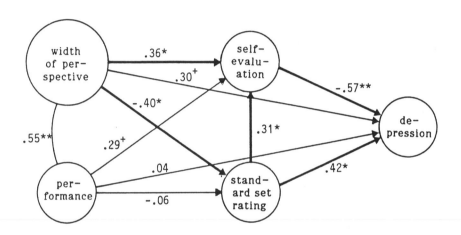

Note.
Only qualified interpretation is possible; cf. text.
n=30.
+p<.10. *p<.05. **p<.01.
beta=.36, t=1.82, p<.05
beta=.30, t=1.35, p<.10
beta=.29, t=1.38, p<.10
beta=-.40, t=-1.91, p<.05
beta=.31, t=1.71, p<.05
beta=-.57, t=-2.86, p<.01
beta=.42, t=2.16, p<.05

FIGURE 4.

No threat conditions. Standardset rating as an additional predictor

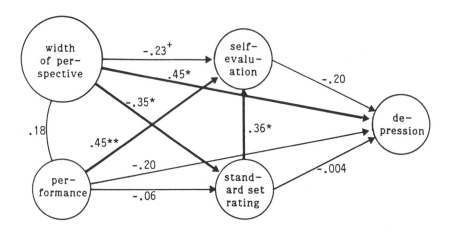

Note.

n=30.

+p<.10. *p<.05. **p<.01.

beta=-.23, t=-1.35, p<.10

beta(performance, self-evaluation)=.45, t=2.81, p<.0

beta(perspective, mood)=.45, t=2.4, p<.05

beta=-.35, t=-1.92, p<.05

beta=.36, t=2.14, p<.05

For all other coefficients t<1.0, n.s

As can be seen from Figures 1. and 2., the wide perspective led to more negative self-evaluations for unthreatened subjects (beta=-.35, t=-2.09, p<.05) but not so for threatened subjects (beta=.17, t=.81, n.s.). If the standard set rating was introduced as an additional predictor (cf. Figure 3.) the beta coefficient between perspective and self-evaluation for threatened subjects reached significance (beta=.36, t=2.14, p<.05). The path between standard set rating and self-evaluation was also significant (beta=.31, t=1.71, p<.05). The standard set rating was a traditional suppressor variable. The variable increased the predictive power of perspective for self-evaluation by suppressing irrelevant variances in the predictor variable 'perspective'. In this special case, the irrelevant variance should have been produced by the confounded effect of performance. The standard set rating variable suppressed that part of the variance which was due to the dependence of self-evaluation on the perspective manipulation. If the effect of the perspective manipulation on self-evaluation was suppressed, the beta coefficient between performance and self-evaluation decreased correspondingly (beta=.29, t=1.38, p<.10). These findings clarify why the coefficients between both exogenous variables and self-evaluation for the threatened subjects did not reach significance in Figure 1.: they both operated in the same direction on the self-evaluation variable. The wider the perspective and the better the performance, the more positive was the self-evaluation. The perspective exerted a paradoxical effect in the threat condition.

Since perspective and performance were correlated, it remains unclear whether the path between perspective and self-evaluation would have reached significance if the variables had been uncorrelated or whether the beta coefficient between performance and self-evaluation would have reached significance. The beta between perspective and self-evaluation became beta=.35 (t=2.01, p<.05) if the predictor 'performance' was excluded from the regression equation. The beta between performance and self-evaluation became beta=.43 (t=-2.5, p<.01) if the predictor 'perspective' was excluded.

Mood was directly influenced by perspectives for unthreatened subjects (beta=.45, t=2.4, p<.05; cf. Figure 2.). This path was only marginally significant (beta=.30, t=1.35, p<.10) in the threat conditions (cf. Figure 1.) but the beta-coefficient was clearly higher as compared to the simple correlation coefficient (r=-.06; cf. Table 5.). Therefore, a suppression effect should have had emanated from either self-evaluation or standard set rating. For identification of the suppressor variable, only two of the multiple predictors were entered into seperate regression analyses. The suppressor effect came from the self-rating variable ($r_{perspective, mood}$=-.06; beta=.09). Such a suppression was absent in the unthreatened groups. Whereas a wide perspective had a direct negative effect on mood for unthreatened subjects (beta=.45, t=2.42, p<.05) the effect of the perspective manipulation on mood was mediated through both self- and standard set-evaluation under threat of self-esteem. Paradoxically, under threat (cf. Figure 3.) a wide perspective (together with better performance, $r_{perspective, performance}$=.55, p<.01) yielded more positive self-evaluations (beta=.36, t=1.81, p<.05) which in turn had a positive effect on mood (beta=-.57, t=-2.86, p<.01). At the same time, a wide perspective led to more negative standard set ratings (beta=-.40, t=-1.91, p<.05) which in turn had a positive effect on mood (beta=.42, t=2.16, p<.05). However, the more negative the standard set rating, the more negative self-evaluation became (beta=.31, t=1.71, p<.05). A negative self-evaluation in turn contributed to negative mood. A suppressor effect emanated from self-evaluation on the path between standard set rating and mood: if only standard set- and self-rating were used as predictors for mood, a beta of .27, t=1.62, p<.10 resulted for the path between standard set rating and mood. The simple intercorrelation between standard set rating and mood was r=.23, n.s. (cf. Table 5.), i.e. the self-rating exerted a suppression effect.

Discussion

Results are in line with the hypothesis that a large perspective with positively shifted origin produces more negative judgments and mood. The effects of the perspective manipulation were quite strong for all dependent variables. Comparisons between expected and observed values, however, revealed that only relative shifts in judgments and mood were dependent on the perspective manipulation. Absolute values could not be predicted. The results did not confirm the hypothesis that reference scales to be used for judgments are built up by anchoring the extremes of a certain stimulus continuum to the extremes of a given response modality (Upshaw, 1969a).

In line with our hypotheses, judgments at the second point of measurement were determined by the parameters of the narrow perspective in the threat conditions. On the other hand, we did not anticipate judgments to be already positively distorted at the first point of measurement, that is to say, when only one perspective was available.

Without threat, subjects did not use the most extreme stimuli either. When two perspectives were made available subjects used a "compromise perspective" of which parameters corresponded to the averaged parameters of the two induced perspectives.

These results are incompatible with Uphsaw's (1969a) prediction. As far as we know, this part of perspective theory has never been tested empirically. In the typical empirical studies on perspective theory, different ranges of stimuli to be used for judgment of a certain stimulus were manipulated between subjects (i.e. Ostrom, 1970; Upshaw, 1978) or it has been shown that subjects extend a given range of stimuli in the direction of their own attitude if the latter is situated outside the range of presented attitude statements (Upshaw, 1962). In our experiment subjects had to solve a more difficult task. They had to integrate two different ranges of stimuli to judge performances. It appears that subjects stored perspectives in memory. If more than one perspective was available, perspectives were integrated. Perspectives could not be activated separately once they were stored in memory. Rather, subjects activated a compromise perspective of which parameters were equivalent to the averaged parameters of all induced perspectives in order to judge a certain stimulus. Hence, possibly the standard set as such was effective as an additional perspective. This would explain why threatened subjects in the narrow-wide condition used a perspective of which the range was even narrower than that of the narrow perspective. This possibility has to be scrutinized further in a second experiment.

In summary, relative shifts in judgments were effectively predicted by the perspective manipulation. Absolute values, however, could not be predicted on the basis of Upshaw's assumption that the most extreme stimuli are used as anchors. From comparison of observed and expected values it could be inferred that subjects integrated the two induced perspectives into a compromise perspective the parameters of which were equivalent to the averaged parameters of the induced perspectives.

As anticipated, the standard set ratings were more positive under threat. At odds with our hypotheses, the more positive means did not correspond with greater standard deviations. Thus, more positive means were not unequivocally the result of subjects' using narrower perspectives. In addition, the anticipated three-way interaction was not significant for any of the dependent variables. The following data pattern should have emerged if threatened subjects would have used only the narrow perspective even if two perspectives were available: judgments were anticipated to become more positive in the wide-narrow condition but to remain stable in the narrow-wide condition for threatened subjects; for unthreatened subjects, on the other hand, judgments and mood were expected to become more negative from time 1 to time 2 in the narrow-wide condition and more positive in the wide-narrow condition. Such a pattern could not be confirmed.

Threatened subjects did not use only the more narrow perspective when two perspectives were available. What is more, judgments were already positively distorted at the first point of measurement. It appears, subjects contrasted their judgments with the lower anchor of the response scale. In other words, subjects end-anchored a stimulus continuum to the response scale which was extended at its lower end. As a result, the range of the response scale used was smaller, leading to smaller dispersions of judgment. Under threat, the lower parts of the response modality were considered inappropriate to judge any of the stimuli. Further support for this interpretation is a general positivity bias in judgments that was present in all groups. This can be seen from the comparison between expected and observed values. In all experimental groups, deviations of observed from expected values were in a positive direction.

The unexpected effects are attributed to the evaluatively negative label of the lower response scale anchor. While instructing the subjects on how to use the response modality, the experimenter had described the lower anchor as "the end where something should be judged

that you think is really bad". Since they were given
negative feedback on own performances, subjects in all
experimental groups were in a situation of an anti-judge
who has to express his attitude on a scale of which the
anti-anchor is evaluatively negative. In previous studies
it has been consistently shown that this leads to less
polarized ratings (Eiser & Mower White, 1974, 1975; Eiser
& van der Pligt, 1982) (cf. Chapter I, pp. 24-30). In our
experiment subjects might have contrasted their judgments away from the evaluatively negative anchor
independently of the perspective manipulation. Under
threat this tendency was even stronger because giving
judgments near a negatively labeled anchor intensified
threat to self-esteem.

Further support for this interpretation is the fact that
the standard set ratings were more positively distorted
than self-evaluations. More positive standard set ratings
occurred because the lower objects were disproportionately overestimated, as is indicated by the negative
skewness of the judgment distribution in all groups. This
tendency was especially strong under threat, which is
reflected in the significantly more negatively skewed
judgment distribution for threatened subjects. It seems
likely that these results were produced by the evaluatively negative labeling of the lower response scale

anchor. Judging near that anchor intensified the threat to self-esteem.

These results contradict perspective theory. From perspective theory one would have expected standard set stimuli to be linearly rated. Specifically, an equal distribution should have resulted from the standard set ratings because objects were equally distant from each other and because they all were "in-range stimuli" (Upshaw, 1962), i.e. they fell within the extremes of both the wide and the narrow perspective. Observed values were at odds with this expectation. In line with our hypotheses, however, a negatively skewed distribution resulted under threat and the distributions were more positively skewed in all experimental groups at the second point of measurement. We have hypothesized that judgments are not only determined by the actual stimulus range but also by prior judgments which have been entered into a person's "life perspective". Since judgments were positively distorted under threat, a more negatively skewed distribution was expected than for the conditions without threat. Overall, negative as compared to positive judgments (relative to the origin of the response scale) were expected to occur more frequently if the perspectives would have been used normatively. Hence, it is in line with our hypotheses that the distribution was more positively skewed at the second point of measurement: prior negative judgments exerted a negative influence on actual judgments beyond the stimulus range. The positive skewness at the second point of measurement is interpreted as indication that actual judgments were entered into the "life perspective". However, our hypotheses were only relatively and not absolutely supported. Given that the normative application of perspectives would have resulted in more frequent negative than positive judgments, we had anticipated a positively skewed distribution at the first point of measurement and a further intensification of this positive skewness for the second point of measurement. This expectation was not met because of the general positivity bias which was due to the evaluatively negative response scale anchor. As a result, negative judgments did not occur more often than positive ones. The skewness was negative at the first point of measurement and only relatively less negative at the second measurement point.

We have interpreted the fact that overestimation of objects decreased within each set of measurements as an effect of previous judgments. The more frequent negative judgments were already given, the more negative actual judgments should be. It might be said, however, that the decrease of overestimation simply reflects the way in which the standard set ratings had been obtained: Judgments of the standard set stimuli were given by means of putting magnets on a metal ledge. Only when the first standard set ratings were finished was the metal ledge exchanged for a new one. Thus, subjects had in front of them a record of their previous judgments. Subjects might therefore have used their own previous judgments as a new frame of reference. Therefore, the decrease in overestimation of stimuli with increasing height of objects might have been an artefact of judgment measurement. This argument has to be examined further in a second experiment.

In summary, our hypothesis that subjects would produce more positive judgments under threat to self-esteem was confirmed. Unexpectedly, this effect was not the result of subjects' using only the narrower of the perspectives provided. Rather, subjects produced positively distorted judgments at the first point of measurement, i.e. when only one perspective was available. In addition, more positive judgments did not coincide with larger dispersions. It appears that subjects in general contrasted their judgments away from the evaluatively negative lower anchor and that this tendency was stronger under threat to self-esteem. The closer the object was to the lower anchor, the more it was positively overestimated. Overall, slightly negative skews in the individual distributions of standard set ratings were obtained in all experimental groups. These distributions were significantly more negatively skewed in the threat conditions. Ratings were influenced by prior judgments in that these distributions were more positively skewed at the second point of measurement. This is interpreted as an indication that judgments were entered into the "life perspective".

In order to interpret the effects of the threat manipulation on self-evaluations and mood, real performances had to be taken into account. Performances were signficantly different between groups. This was not anticipated: no differences in experimental manipulations were present up to that point in time when subjects had produced their performances. Thus, the differences in performance may have been due to experimenter influences. The subjects in the "threat, wide-narrow condition" performed significantly better. This condition can be conceived of as the "most threatening one". Not only because the confederate's superiority was emphasized (threat manipulation) but also because the confederate's supposed performance provided the wide perspective (through the order manipulation). Possibly, the experimenter may have "felt sorry" for the subjects in this condition and, as a result, reinforced them nonverbally during their play what may have led to the significantly better performances.

That no significant main effect of the threat-manipulation on self-evaluation and mood was found may have been due to the significant performance differences. Possibly, main effects were destroyed by an interaction between threat and order manipulation. Self-evaluations were more positive in the wide-narrow condition under threat than without threat but more negative in the narrow-wide condition. However, this may simply reflect the significantly better performance under threat in the wide-narrow condition.

Results were not completely parallel for self-evaluation and mood. The marginally significant main effect of the threat manipulation was due to more <u>positive</u> self-evaluations. This was different for mood. A marginally significant main effect of threat on mood occurred that was due to more <u>negative</u> mood in the threat condition if the effects of self-evaluations on mood were controlled. It seems as if the threat manipulation was effective in opposite directions for self-evaluations and mood, respectively. Negative effects of the threat manipulation on mood were prevented by positive self-evaluations.

Due to the significant performance differences between groups a complete causal structure model could not be computed to further scrutinize these results. Separate structural models were tested for both the threat and the no-threat conditions. These analyses confirmed that, under threat, self-evaluations were "used" to prevent situational depression. Whereas for unthreatened subjects a wide perspective led to more negative standard set ratings and self-evaluations and to more negative mood, for the threatened subjects the negative effect of perspective on mood was suppressed by positively distorted self-evaluations. Apparently, judgments had an effect on mood if and only if self-esteem threat was given. Without threat, judgments were dependent on the perspective manipulation but judgments in turn did not have any effect on mood.

These results have implications for the concept of congeneric scales (Upshaw, 1978). For Upshaw, a change in stimulus perception can be assumed if and only if shifts in judgments are present on different congeneric scales which are intercorrelated and uninfluenced by any perspective manipulation. Our results showed that, only under certain conditions, the internal representation of a self-produced outcome as a latent variable was linearly transformed into different response modalities. The outcome was simultaneously reflected in standard set ratings, self-evaluations, and mood ratings if no threat was present. Under threat, on the other hand, judgments not only served a communicative function. Rather, they had effects on mood as such. This implies that self-relevant judgments may be positively distorted in order to satisfy a self-protection motive. As mood is improved through positive self-ratings, the stimulus may even be seen as more positive in retrospect.

Upshaw's functional criterion for a change in stimulus perception (Upshaw, 1978) was clearly met for the unthreatened subjects. Perspective-dependent shifts were present for standard set ratings, self-evaluations, and mood rating while no mood related perspective manipulation was given. The scales were intercorrelated (though for standard set ratings and mood only marginally significant so, cf. Table 5.).

For the threatened subjects, however, only self-evaluation and mood were significantly intercorrelated. Perspective-dependent shifts appeared with respect to the judgment variables only, and these in turn had effects on mood. The wide perspective led to more negative standard set ratings and at the same time to more positive self-evaluations. The judgment pattern for threatened subjects can be interpreted as a self-protection mechanism. Positively distorted self-evaluations as well as negative standard set ratings suppressed a negative effect of perceived failure on mood. The finding that positively distorted self-evaluations improved mood supports the assumption that self-serving biases are emotionally functional (cf. Snyder et al., 1976; Harvey &

Weary, 1981; Boski, 1983). The standard set outcomes were introduced to the subjects as plays of other anonymous persons. For this reason, the relationship between negative standard set ratings and improved mood might suggest that putting down others might be functional for maintaining positive self-esteem (cf. Brewer & Campbell, 1976; Taylor & Doria, 1981; Wills, 1981; Tesser & Campbell, 1982; Bornewasser, 1985). Nevertheless, in our experiments, the standard for self-evaluation increased at the same time as standard set ratings became more negative. The more negative the standard set judgments, the more negative self-ratings became, and this in turn had a negative effect on mood. Apparently, standard set judgments had a direct and a mediated effect on mood. Possibly, these results reflect different judgment patterns between subjects: whereas some of the subjects used the perspectives to judge both standard set objects and own performances, others might have used the perspectives for the standard set ratings only.

To conclude, results of the first experiment were in line with our hypotheses. Judgments and mood were dependent on experimental perspectives and judgments were more positive under threat. Contrary to our hypotheses, more positive judgments were not due to the use of the narrower perspective. Rather, subjects contrasted their judgments from the evaluatively negative response anchor, especially under threat. It appears that the threatened subjects considered the lower part of the response scale as inappropriate for judgments of any of the stimuli.

As expected, a more positively skewed distribution emerged at the second measurement point.

Relative shifts but not absolute values of judgments and mood could be predicted from Upshaw's assumption that people use the two most extreme stimuli to form a perspective. It appears that available perspectives were integrated into a "compromise perspective". Therefore the standard set as such might have been effective as an additional perspective. Thus, for all judgments following the first standard set rating, effects of perspectives and of the standard set as such might have been confounded.

Causal structures were mainly in line with our expectations. Due to significant performance differences between groups, however, the effects of perspective manipulation and performance were confounded. Hence, our interpretations of the causal structures are preliminary.

Experiment II

This experiment tests the same hypotheses as Experiment I, but with some improvements to the procedure.

Method

Subjects

Again, subjects were 60 male adolescents. Subjects were between 14 and 25 years of age. They were paid 20 German marks for participation in the two-hour experimental session.

Stimulus materials

The stimulus materials used were identical to those in Experiment I.

Procedure

The procedure was identical to that in Experiment I aside from the following differences.

To rule out significant performance differences the experimenter was blind to experimental condition up to that point in time of the experimental session when the plays of the subjects were completed. Therefore the confederate took care about all necessary preparations and deposited a card with the condition written on it at a prearranged location.

In order to clarify whether the threat manipulation had an effect only because of the evaluatively negative response scale anchor, a neutral response scale labeling was used. The lower scale anchor was explained by the experimenter as "the end where something should be judged that you think is really low".

The standard set was shown only once, namely at the end of the experimental session, in order to rule out any effects of the standard set rating on following judgments. An additional self-evaluation was measured immediately after the standard set rating in order to examine further the effect of the standard set judgments. Moreover, for half of the subjects, this third self-evaluation was measured on a different instrument (modality manipulation) in order to find out whether a possible effect of the standard set rating would not carry over to another instrument.

To rule out the possibility that subjects used their previous judgments as a frame of reference, the measurement instrument was changed in the following manner. An electric mechanism was applied to the metal ledge that allowed for an immediate measurement of a given rating. An electric circuit was closed at that point where the magnet was put on the ledge. The resulting resistor was indicated on an ammeter. Subjects were given one magnet only which had to be removed from the ledge immediately after it had been positioned.

Dependent measures

These were identical to those in Experiment I, the only difference being that standard set ratings were only measured once and self-evaluations were measured three times.

Results

Task performance data

Again, a two-way ANOVA computed on performances showed significant differences between groups. Threatened subjects performed significantly poorer ($F_{(1,56)}=9.29$, $p=.003$).

Effects of threat to self-esteem

Analysis of variance for repeated measures (2x2x2) was computed on the self-evaluations which were measured immediately after the perspective inductions. There was no main effect of the threat manipulation on self-evaluations ($F_{(1,56)}$=2.52, p=.114). However, only within-subjects effects could be interpreted because of the significant performance differences: a significant interaction between threat manipulation and time of measurement was obtained. Whereas self-evaluations remained the same from time 1 to time 2 for threatened subjects, they became more negative for unthreatened subjects ($F_{(1,56)}$=4.67, p=.033). A three-way interaction for threat manipulation, order of perspective induction, and time of measurement was marginally significant ($F_{(1,56)}$=3.51, p=.063). For the unthreatened subjects in the wide-narrow condition, self-evaluations became more positive from time 1 to time 2 and became more negative to the same extent in the narrow-wide condition. However, for threatened subjects self-evaluations became more positive from time 1 to time 2 but not more negative in the narrow-wide condition.

Analysis of variance for repeated measures on mood scores showed no main effect of the threat manipulation either (F < 1). A significant interaction between threat and time of measurement was found ($F_{(1,56)}$=4.3, p=.04). Whereas mood was stable over the two measurement points for threatened subjects, mood worsened for the unthreatened subjects.

For the standard set rating, no effect of the threat manipulation was found, neither on mean judgments ($F_{(1,56)}=1.16$, n.s.) nor on standard deviations ($F_{(1,56)}=1.57$, n.s.). A significant main effect on the degree of skew appeared ($F_{(1,56)}=4.12$, p=.044). The skewness was more negative for threatened subjects.

Effects of perspectives

Analysis of variance for repeated measures on self-evaluations yielded a significant interaction between order of perspective induction and time of measurement ($F_{(1,56)}=24.43$, p<.001). Specifically, when the wide perspective was induced first, self-evaluations became more positive from time 1 to time 2. The opposite held true when the narrow perspective was induced first.

For mood scores, the same analysis yielded a corresponding significant interaction effect ($F_{(1,56)}=10.054$, p=.002). Whereas mood was more negative at time 1 if the wide perspective was induced first the opposite was true for the narrow-wide conditions. In addition, a significant main effect for time of measurement was found ($F_{(1,56)}=6.35$, p=.014). Mood deteriorated from time 1 to time 2.

Effects of standard set rating

Analysis of variance for repeated measures was performed on self-evaluations which were measured immediately before and after the standard set rating. Subjects were grouped according to experimental conditions. The only significant effect was an interaction between order of perspective induction and time of measurement $(F_{(1,56)}=7.3$, $p=.008)$. Whereas in the wide-narrow conditions self-evaluations were more negative after the standard set ratings, the opposite held true for the narrow-wide groups. A two-way analysis of variance for the third self-evaluation did not render any differences between experimental groups $(F_{(1,56)}=1.15$, $p=.29$ for threat; $F_{(1,56)}=.303$, n.s. for order of perspective induction).

For half of the subjects, self-evaluations were measured on a second instrument at the third point of measurement. Subjects were grouped with respect to the modality manipulation and with respect to order of perspective induction. Analysis of variance for repeated measures yielded no other effects aside from the interaction effect between order of induction and time (see above; $F_{(1,56)}=7.14$, $p=.009)$.

Comparison between expected and observed values

For self-evaluations, tests between expected and observed values showed that unthreatened subjects used the induced perspective at the first point of measurement ($t=0.83$, $p<.30$ for wide-narrow condition; $t=-0.91$, $p<.30$ for narrow-wide condition). Threatened subjects, however, gave more negative ratings than would have been expected from using the induced perspectives. A hypothetical perspective with a range of $x=34.7$ would explain the observed values in the "threat, wide-narrow condition". Such a hypothetical perspective produces marginally significantly more negative values than would have had the induced one, namely the wide perspective with a range of $x=30$ ($t=-1.38$, $p<.10$ for comparison between observed and expected values). Subjects in the "threat, narrow- wide condition" used a perspective with a range of $x=22.44$. Again, resulting values were significantly more negative than the expected ones ($t=-2.89$, $p<.05$).

At the second point of measurement, subjects in both wide-narrow conditions used the compromise perspective between the two induced ones ($t=0.54$, $p=.50$ for threatened subjects; $t=0.08$, $p=.50$ for unthreatened subjects). Threatened subjects in the narrow-wide condition used a perspective which, in terms of range, lay between the large perspective actually induced and the compromise perspective ($t=1.96$, $p<.10$, and $t=-1.35$, $p<.10$, respectively). Unthreatened subjects in the narrow-wide condition used a perspective that was even wider than the wide one (range=40.7). Observed values were significantly more negative than expected ones (t=-2.85, p<.05).

Self-evaluations at the third point of measurement were best described by a compromise perspective between the two experimentally induced ones. t-values for tests between observed and expected values of the compromise perspective were as follows:
- t=0.29, p=.50 for "threat, wide-narrow condition";
- t=0.91, p<.30 for "threat, narrow-wide condition";
- t=1.94, p<.10 for "no threat, wide-narrow condition" and
- t=0.61, p=.50 for "no threat, narrow-wide condition".

Mood scores were transformed into standard T-scores before they were tested against expected values. Overall, observed values were clearly below the expected ones. According to the procedure in Experiment I, expected values were computed for a response scale that was constricted to the lower two thirds of the original range. Again, at the first point of measurement, observed values were definitely below expected ones thus rendering a significance-testing superfluous. At the second point of measurement, values in the wide-narrow conditions were in accordance with expected values of the perspective actually induced (t=1.71, p<.20 for threatened subjects; t=0.66, p=.50 for unthreatened subjects). In addition, values in the "no threat, narrow-wide condition" corresponded to expected ones (t=-1.72, p<.20).

The results of Experiment I led us to believe that the standard set as such might have functioned as an additional perspective. For this reason, observed values for the standard set ratings, which had been obtained after induction of both the wide and the narrow perspective, were tested against expected values from the following two hypothetical perspectives:

- compromise perspective between wide and narrow perspective;
- compromise perspective between wide and narrow perspective and the standard set as a perspective.

Observed values were better described by the expected values of the compromise perspective between wide, narrow and standard set (t=0.94, p<.30) than by the compromise perspective between wide and narrow (t=5.41, p<.01).

Causal structures

Causal links between variables for a specified model are to be estimated from the sample covariance matrix. The prerequisite, that variables are intercorrelated was not met, however. Pearson product-moment coefficients between self-evaluation and mood were not significant ($r=-.08$, n.s. for time 1; $r=-.16$, n.s. for time 2). Therefore no causal models were specified.

Chapter 3

General Discussion

Effects of threat to self-esteem

In Experiment II no significant main effect of the threat manipulation was found in the analyses of variance. This might have been due to the significant performance differences. It is difficult to explain why threatened subjects performed significantly more poorly. The reason does not seem to be either the experimental manipulations or experimenter influences. Comparisons between expected and observed values that take performance differences into account revealed that threatened subjects gave more negative judgments of their own performances. No further results were obtained from these comparisons for mood: absolute values could not be explained by any of the hypothetical perspectives. Rather, mood was rated more positively than would have been predicted from manipulated perspectives in all experimental groups.

To summarize, the threat manipulation had a much weaker effect in the second experiment. In addition, the effects in the two experiments were in opposite directions. Whereas threatened subjects in Experiment I showed more positively biased judgments, the opposite held true in Experiment II.

We started out from the idea that threat is a situational factor leading to the greater use of a self-protective perspective. In particular, we assumed that threatened subjects would exclusively use the narrow perspective if both perspectives were available.

This hypothesis could not be confirmed. In the first experiment, positive self-evaluations did not correspond with larger dispersions and threatened subjects gave distorted judgments already at the first point of measurement. In addition, effects of the threat manipulation were in opposite directions in both experiments. The manipulation check did not reveal exactly <u>how</u> the threat manipulation had the effect which it did. The post-experimental questionnaire only asked whether the threat manipulation had been convincing ("Do you remember what level your partner has achieved in the game?"; if subjects had believed in the threat induction, they should remember the level that the confederate had supposedly reached). As expected, threatened subjects remembered their partner's performance result better than did the unthreatened subjects (Chi²-test). However, our results seem to indicate that the effect of threat was more complex. Possibly, the effect of the threat manipulation has been mediated by different intervening variables which may be responsible for the opposite effects in the two experiments. The following differences between the experiments can be specified:

- Unavoidably, experimenter and confederate were more practised in the second experiment.
- The order in which the different measures were obtained in the experimental session was different: in the first experiment, self-evaluations were measured immediately after the standard set measurement. In the second experiment, self-evaluation measures were taken immediately after the perspective induction.
- In the first experiment, the lower anchor of the response scale was labeled in an evaluatively negative way by the experimenter. In the second experiment, the response scale was connotatively neutral.

These differences may have caused the dissimilar effects of the threat manipulation in one of the following ways.
- The degree of experienced threat was different in the two experiments and intensity of threat was non-linearly related to self-evaluations.
- The direction of the threat effect depended on additional intervening variables. Thus, either
  - threat may have increased the sensitivity of stimulus discrimination and/or influenced the response criterion for different judgments. Depending on additional variables, namely the different order in which the measures were obtained and the different response language, judgments were biased in a

positive or negative direction <u>at the level of response;</u>
and/or

- threat may have influenced the achievement motivation. Depending on different response languages either success or failure orientation may have been induced.

Could threat and self-evaluation be non-linearly related? The relationship between threat and self-evaluations might possibly be described by an inverted u-shaped function (Berlyne, 1960). It is conceivable that subjects do not show any self-serving biases if the degree of experienced threat is very high. If this were the case, results should have been similar for nonthreatened and highly threatened subjects. In fact, the threatened subjects in the second (but not the first) experiment responded similarly to non-threatened subjects (who did not differ between the two experiments). This might suggest that threat was more intense in the second experiment. However, this does not seem plausible at all, for reasons of the different labeling of the response scale and the fact that both experimenter and confederate had much more practice, probably resulting in a more relaxed athmosphere. Therefore, if anything, threat should have been <u>less</u> intense in the second experiment.

Hence, the different effects cannot be explained with a non-linear relationship between degree of experienced threat and self-evaluations.

Were there differences in sensitivity and/or response bias?

Perhaps judgment biases were not due to the fact that threatened subjects used different perspectives but rather to a process which was effective at the level of response. Under threat, the relatively lower performance result of the subject was emphasized. Therefore it can be assumed that heightened awareness, which influences stimulus discriminability, resulted from increased self-focussing. In other words, threat to self-esteem might have had a nonspecific effect in the sense that it contributed to better stimulus discrimiation. Upmeyer (1981) conceives of the self as a trigger of attention.

"... we should like to introduce and discuss a distinction which can be used in partitioning information into more and less relevant classes. This is the concept of the self widely employed in social psychology... Incoming information is thought to be checked by the individual with respect to evaluative content about the self. (...) The conception of the self presented here has its roots in Darwinian thinking. Dangers and challenges as well as the desire for security render self-relevant information more important and thus more salient than information concerning objects and events which are irrelevant to the self" (p. 269).

As a result, stimulus discrimination of self-relevant information is improved. When a perceived stimulus is pictured into a response modality other variables might come into effect depending on which judgments may be positively or negatively distorted. Upmeyer (1981, 1982) distinguishes between sanctions, expectations (because of the stimulus frequency) and correspondences as possible determinants of response tendencies. Sanctions can consist of anticipated negative consequences supposed that the response is _not_ distorted or in positive consequences in the case of a biased response.

According to this interpretation sanctions were effective in both our experiments. In the first experiment negative consequences were to be expected from unbiased judgments, and in the second experiment positive consequences could be expected from negatively distorted judgments.

Why were negative consequences to be expected from unbiased judgments in the first experiment?
In Experiment I, the negative connotation of the lower response scale anchor may have had a similar effect to that of a sanction (Upmeyer, 1981). Judgments were contrasted with the lower anchor because an unbiased response would have led to negative consequences for the subjects, namely to a negative effect on mood, reflecting

negative self-evaluations. This assumption is supported by the results of the path analyses. For threatened subjects, negative self-evaluations had negative effects on mood. Under threat, a desire to judge one's own performance positively was intensified. This was because positive self-evaluations helped prevent a negative effect of negative outcome representation on mood.

Why were positive consequences to be expected from negatively distorted judgments in the second experiment?

Aside from the change of response language, the order in which the measures were obtained was changed in the second experiment: self-evaluations were given immediately after induction of a perspective. Since the experimenter was present a strong demand characteristic (Orne, 1962) to use the perspectives in a normative fashion might have been operating. Social desirability (Edwards, 1957) might have led subjects to underestimate their performances, thus acknowledging their own inferiority and the confederate's superiority. This tendency may have been intensified under threat because here the inferiority of the subject was emphasized by the experimenter. Hence, positive consequences (i.e. social recognition by the experimenter) could have been anticipated as a result of negatively distorted (or 'modest') judgments. In addition, no negative consequences were to be expected from negative self-ratings as was the case in Experiment I: self-ratings and mood were not correlated in Experiment II.

To what extent do our empirical results fit these interpretations?

If threat was effective at the level of response, this would explain why positively distorted judgments did not coincide with larger dispersions: threat did not have an effect on the internal representation of outcomes (which corresponds to dispersions) but only had an effect at the level of response.

Originally, we had expected interactive effects between threat and perspective manipulation as indication of changed outcome representation. These effects were not obtained in the first experiment but only in Experiment II: whereas without threat self-evaluations and mood became more negative from time 1 to time 2, they remained stable under threat. The expected three-way interaction was marginally significant for self-evaluations. Specifically, ratings became more positive from time 1 to time 2 in the wide-narrow condition but not more negative in the narrow-wide condition under conditions of threat. Without threat, however, ratings became more negative in the narrow-wide condition to the same extent

as they became more positive in the wide-narrow
condition.

These effects support our hypotheses which could not be
confirmed in Experiment I. We have assumed that
interaction effects were not found in the first experiment because of the evaluatively negative response scale
anchor which led to positively biased judgments in all
experimental groups, i.e. also at the first point of
measurement. Interactions were found in the second
experiment in which the response modality was neutral.
Results seem to indicate that threat led to a self-protective selection of perspectives.

How can this interpretation be reconciled with the
interpretation that threat had an effect at the level of
response? Comparisons between expected and observed
values showed that interactions in Experiment II were
due to the fact that negative distortions under threat
were eliminated at the second point of measurement.
That is to say, the interactive effects reflect a process
at the response level as well. Whereas at the first point
of measurement, i.e. when only one perspective was
available, negatively distorted judgments seemed socially
desirable, at the second point of measurement no demand
characteristic to use a certain perspective was present.

As a result, no positive consequences were to be anticipated from negative distortion of judgments.

To summarize, our hypothesis that threat would lead to the exclusive use of the narrow perspective was not confirmed. Since threat led to opposite effects in both experiments it was assumed that threat had a nonspecific effect on judgments. Possibly, threat led to better stimulus discrimination. Depending on additional variables (in this case particularly sanctions; Upmeyer, 1981), positive or negative response biases could have occurred. In Experiment I, anticipation of negative mood as an effect of self-evaluation near the evaluatively negative lower anchor of the response modality led to positively distorted judgments in the threat conditions. No such distortion was found for unthreatened subjects because here negative self-evaluations had no effects on mood. In Experiment II, self-evaluations were given immediately after perspective induction. In the threat conditions the confederate's superiority was emphasized by the experimenter. Hence, positive consequences, i.e. social recognition by the experimenter, could have been expected from negatively biased self-ratings. In addition, no negative consequences were to be expected from negative self-evaluations: judgments and mood were uncorrelated. This, again, might have been due to the evaluatively neutral response scale for self-evaluations.

Interactive effects between perspective manipulations and threat in Experiment II could have been due to the fact that no positive consequences of negatively distorted judgments were to be anticipated at the second point of measurement. These effects were consistent with our original hypothesis that threat leads to self-protective perspective selection.

Note that anticipated affects are conceived of as 'sanctions' that may influence response generation (Upmeyer, 1981). Such a view is in line with our results that judgments not only served a communicative but also an emotion-regulatory function. That is to say, positively distorted judgments help maintain feelings of positive well-being.

Could threat have influenced achievement motivation?
An alternative explanation is that threat had a nonspecific effect by increasing achievement motivation; depending on the provided response scale, this effect may have had a more specific direction. So far we have presupposed
- that the response language did not have an effect on

the internal stimulus representation but was only effective at the level of response;
- that the available perspective could be reduced in width only at its upper end. In other words, an extention of the upper anchor was assumed to be impossible and the lower anchor was assumed to be fixed.

Possibly both assumptions have to be rejected. It is conceivable that response language and the threat manipulation interacted: under threat, the internally represented stimulus continuum may have been influenced by the response language, but not so when threat was absent.

In both experiments the threat manipulation involved the emphasizing of the confederate's superiority. Therefore, one can assume that achievement motivation was higher under threat because competition was induced. That is to say, threatened subjects in both experiments should have been more concerned with possible performance results, i.e. with possible success or failure. It is conceivable that the threat manipulation induced fear of failure in the first experiment and hope for success in the second one.

In the first experiment, subjects were instructed to judge an outcome which they considered really bad at the lower end of the response scale. This might have led subjects to think of a much more negative event than the presumed lower anchor (failure at the first level of the computer game). The threat manipulation may have suggested the possibility of even more abject failure. Subjects might have thought about the possibility that they would be unable to handle the joystick, that the experimenter would interrupt their play because they were playing too poorly, or such like. In other words, if the lower anchor of the perceptual continuum had been manipulated, threatened subjects would have been expected to use an even poorer performance to end-anchor the evaluatively negative extreme of the response scale. However, the lowest performance outcome was (necessarily) held constant since the plays all had to start from the very beginning of the game. Therefore, this hypothesis cannot be tested directly.

Such an interpretation would account for the unexpected result that more positive judgments under threat did not correspond to larger dispersions. Under threat, the perspectives were not only constricted at the upper anchor but at the same time extended at the lower end. In addition, such an interpretation would explain why, unexpectedly, threatened subjects biased judgments to a greater extent than one would expect if they were just using the narrow perspective. They showed positively distorted judgments at the first time of measurement, i.e.

when only one perspective was available, by "imagina-
tively" expanding the perceptual continuum at its lower
end.

If the negative response language led subjects to extend
their perceptual perspective at its lower end, the general
positivity bias which was present in all experimental
groups in Experiment I is explained. Subjects were in the
situation of an anti-judge in a P+-condition (cf. Eiser &
van der Pligt, 1982) since all subjects were given failure
feedback. That is to say, own scale position and connotative meaning of the response scale were evaluatively
inconsistent. As a result, a general positivity effect
occurred (cf. Eiser & Mower White, 1974; Eiser & Osmon,
1978).

In the second experiment, on the other hand, the
response scale was connotatively neutral. Therefore,
subjects should not have thought about a more negative
outcome than the presumed lower anchor of failure on
the first level of the game.

However, it remains to be explained why a negative
evaluation bias occurred in the second experiment.

It can be assumed that, ordinarily, subjects play at the
computer in hope for success. The newspaper advertisement by means of which subjects were recruited mentioned that computer games were to be played. Presuma-

bly, the sample consisted of subjects who were oriented towards successful achievement in computer games. Since no negative response language was provided, subjects should not have been so concerned with the possibility of failure. Under threat, the confederate's superiority was emphasized. Possibly this led subjects to imagine a game level which was even <u>above</u> the one the confederate had reached thereby extending the perceptual continuum at its upper end. Subjects may have been success-oriented in the second experiment, in the sense of imagining a game level at which they would have had outperformed the confederate. This interpretation is supported by the results of the comparison of expected and observed values. Threatened subjects especially showed a tendency to underestimate their own performances, i.e. they used perspectives which were extended at the upper end.

It is important to note that the terms success- or failure- orientation are not used in their original meaning (Atkinson, 1957). Traditionally, the terms stem from a concept of expectancy which implies that ambiguous stimuli are interpreted consistently with the person's predominant motivational orientation as either positive or negative. That is to say, outcome evaluations are supposedly assimilated to the motivational orientation (cf. Fitch, 1970; Stroebe, 1977). As used here, however, success- and failure-orientation are assumed to lead to contrast effects. If the possibility of complete failure is brought to mind by means of an evaluatively negative response language, the internal stimulus continuum is extended at its lower end and, as a result, outcome evaluations are contrasted from the lower anchor. Therefore, more positive evaluations result in the context of failure-orientation and more negative evaluations in the context of success-orientation. In our approach, the equivalent of a person's motivational orientation is the frequency distribution on his or her life perspective which operates like an expectation. Under uncertainty, outcome evaluations are distorted in direction of the highest density of the distribution (cf. Upmeyer, 1981).

Originally, we assumed that the response language as such would have no effect on the internally represented perspective. We have interpreted results from studies on accentuation (which show less polarization when judges' attitudes and the provided response language are inconsistent) as indication of subjects' reluctance to use the response scale offered to them. However, our results do not support this assumption. It seems that different ranges of stimuli were used as a frame of reference, depending on connotative aspects of the response language. In Eiser and van der Pligt's (1982) terms, our subjects considered different ranges of outcomes as 'appropriate', depending on the response language provided. More precisely, in the first experiment our subjects considered the response scale to be more appropriate for the judgment of a stimulus range with a lower origin than that in the second experiment. For Eiser and van der Pligt (1982), this does not imply that subjects had different perceptual perspectives. The 'appropriate range' does not necessarily equal the range of internally represented stimuli. The 'appropriate range' rather corresponds to the range of outcomes which a certain judge considers may be suitably described by means of a given response scale. However, here it is assumed that the internal representation of an outcome is dependent on the total range of internally represented stimuli, i.e. changes in perspectives correspond to changes in stimulus representation. In more concrete terms, it is inferred that the response language created expectations of the range of possible outcomes.

Such an interpretation is supported by the results of two experiments conducted by Schwarz, Hippler, Deutsch and Strack (1985). The authors supposed that response categories serve an informative function since they teach the judge about the range of possible responses or about the researcher's expectations of responses. Hence, the range of response categories provided is used as a frame of reference to judge own attitudes or behaviors. Mean response categories are considered as representative of usual and extreme categories as representative of unusual attitudes or behaviors. In other words, mean response categories are used like a social comparison standard. Schwarz et al. (1985) manipulated the range of response categories offered to subjects in terms of which to evaluate their own daily use of television. As expected, subjects who where provided with a low range of possible response categories indicated less use of TV and conceived of TV as more important in their lifes. That is to say, estimates of television watching were dependent on assumptions about normal levels inferred from the range of provided response categories. In addition, the lower range produced a contrast effect in the estimation of the importance of TV in one's own life. The own level of use was recognized as above social comparison standards and, as a result, a higher importance was inferred (Experiment I). On the other hand, subjects with the low response scale range were less satisfied with the variety of their leisure time activities (Experiment II). These subjects conceived of less daily use to be usual as compared to subjects who where offered a high response range and as compared to a control group.

With respect to our experiments, Schwarz et al.'s (1985) results show that the response language may activate a stimulus range at the level of internal representation which functions as a frame of reference. The social comparison standard in Schwarz et al.'s (1985) experiments corresponds to the standard for self-evaluations in our studies. If an evaluatively negative response scale was provided a range of possible outcomes with lower origin was activated at the level of internal representation and, as a result, more positive self-evaluations occurred.

To summarize, threat had a nonspecific effect on self-evaluations. This could take the form of threat leading to heightened awareness and hence to improved stimulus discrimination and to judgments being distorted in a positive or negative direction depending on expected sanctions (Upmeyer, 1981). Alternatively, threat may have increased achievement orientation and hence success- or failure-orientation may have been induced depending on aspects of the response language.

These two possibilities cannot be chosen between empirically in the absence of an appropriate manipulation check. An unequivocal interpretation of the threat effect would only be possible if response language and threat were manipulated independently in a further experiment.

Effects of perspectives

Effects of perspectives were quite strong in both experiments and for all dependent variables. However, only relative shifts but not absolute values of judgment and mood could be predicted from Upshaw's assumption that the most extreme stimuli serve as anchors of a judgmental perspective. In both experiments it was found that subjects used a compromise perspective between the two induced ones at the second point of measurement. On the basis of our empirical results, the following elaborations of perspective theory are suggested. Through these, not only relative, but (at least under certain conditions) absolute judgment values may conceivably be predicted:

- People store anchor stimuli of available perspectives.
- If and only if just one perspective is available, and no threat to self-esteem is given in terms of situational aspects or aspects of the response modality, absolute values of judgments can be predicted.
- Several perspectives are integrated in memory. If a certain stimulus is to be judged, a perspective is activated from memory of which the parameters equal the averaged parameters of <u>all</u> relevant perspectives that have been induced up to that point in time.
- Relative shifts in judgments as effects of anchor manipulations can be predicted even if perspectives which are already stored in memory are unknown and

if aspects of threat and evaluative meaning of response modality are left unregarded. Induction of a wide perspective with a higher origin always produces more negative mean judgments and larger standard deviations than the induction of a small perspective with a lower origin.

The standard set as a method

Comparisons between self-evaluations before and after the standard set ratings in Experiment II showed that, only after the standard set ratings had been made, both experimental perspectives became integrated with each other. There was a significant interaction between order of perspective induction (wide-narrow versus narrow-wide) and point of measurement for self-evaluations (before versus after the standard set ratings). This was due to the fact that self-evaluations were dependent on the actual perspective at the second point of measurement. Specifically, judgments were more positive if the narrow perspective was the one actually induced but more negative if the wide perspective was induced. These differences were not present at the third point of measurement. This was also the case for subjects who gave their self-evaluations after the standard set ratings on another instrument. Subjects all gave their judgments on the basis of a compromise perspective between the

two induced ones, and this effect was not modality-
dependent. It seems, an induced perspective is predomi-
nantly in effect for a certain amount of time. Thereafter,
the perspective is integrated with prior perspectives
which are already stored in memory. If a judgment is to
be given, an integrated perspective of which the
parameters equal the averaged parameters of all stored
perspectives is used.

Whereas in both experiments it could be shown that after
the standard set ratings (i.e. for self-evaluations) both
experimental perspectives were used, in the second
experiment empirical ratings of the standard set stimuli
as such were best described by a compromise perspective
between the two experimental ones and the standard set
perspective. That is to say, mean judgments were more
positive and standard deviations were larger for the
standard set ratings than would have been expected if a
compromise perspective between wide and narrow had
been used. The only difference between standard set
ratings and following ratings was that the standard set
ratings were computed on a series of stimuli. Possibly,
frequency effects have to be taken into account to
explain the observed standard set ratings. More precisely,
the normative application of experimental perspectives
would have led to the use of a rather small range as
compared to the whole range of the response scale.

Subjects seemed to use a wider range of the response scale for the standard set rating. This interpretation is consistent with the range-frequency principle (Parducci, 1965). People tend to use a given number of response categories with equal frequency. As a result, it appeared as if standard set ratings were best described by a normative perspective which was wider and had a more positive origin than the compromise perspective between the two induced ones. However, this result is misleading. In fact, observed values are best predicted by a compromise perspective between wide and narrow. In addition, if not a single stimulus but a set of stimuli is to be judged, the freqency principle has to be taken into account.

In summary, relative effects of perspectives can be shown for single stimuli as well as for a set of stimuli. If absolute values are to be predicted, on the other hand, these values can be inferred from a compromise perspective of all perspectives that have been induced up to that point in time with regard to single stimuli only. If a series of stimuli, like the standard set, is to be judged, the frequency principle comes into effect. People tend to cover the whole range of available response categories in judging a series of stimuli.

Scale effects versus changed stimulus-perception
Perspective-dependent effects could be shown in both experiments. Self-evaluation and mood (and standard set ratings in Experiment I; not tested for the influence of perspective in Experiment II) were more negative if the wide perspective was given as compared to when the narrow perspective was given. Nevertheless, mood and self-evaluations were not intercorrelated in Experiment II. This contradicts our expectation that self-evaluations and mood would either both change corresponding to experimental manipulations or that changes in self-evaluations would occur as a result of experimental manipulations which in turn would influence mood. It appears that different groups of subjects were responsible for the effects in the second experiment. Either subjects responded to experimental manipulations with corresponding self-evaluations or with corresponding mood changes.

How are these results to be interpreted in the light of the concept of congeneric scales (Upshaw, 1978)? Upshaw's functional criterion for a change in stimulus-perception was clearly met in Experiment I. In the second experiment, perspective-dependent shifts were present on both self-evaluative and mood scales but scales were not intercorrelated. It could be argued that effects are nothing but scale effects. In opposition to this, we infer that changes in stimulus representation occurred in both experiments because of the following reasons:

- Upshaw (1978) specifies that shifts are to be shown on a scale to which no perspective manipulation directly pertains. In both our experiments no mood-related manipulation was given.

- If mood shifts were scale effects subjects would have had to end-anchor the mood scale with the extreme stimuli of the wide and narrow perspective, respectively. However, in our case, an inventory was used that consisted of a number of single statements which were unweightedly computed into a general depression score. Statements were the same with respect to the extent to which aquiescence represented negative or positive mood. Hence, it was impossible for subjects to end-anchor the extreme stimuli of the response scale to the extremes of the perceptual perspective.

- Mood is the one operationalization of performance perception which is most closely linked to the perceptual level itself.

- A personal reference scale between mood states and verbal expressions used to communicate these states can be assumed. We maintain that such a personal reference scale is used in a relatively stable manner. This is because an internal stimulus continuum of mood states is constricted by the extreme mood states a person has experienced in his or her life.

Because of these reasons we assume that observed changes in mood are necessary and sufficient grounds for inferring a different representation of a self-produced performance outcome, if possible suppression effects of self-evaluations are taken into account. This implies that those subjects who showed perspective-dependent changes in self-evaluations but not in mood in the second experiment were only showing a 'scale' effect (i.e. an effect at the level of verbal response). They fulfilled the experimental task to judge outcomes in a manner that was relative to the perspective presented, but their internal outcome representation was unchanged. As a result, no effects on mood occurred.

A criterion to separate subjects who produced scale effects from those that showed changes in mood could not be found. Following the original distinction between scale and attitude effects (Ostrom & Upshaw, 1968; Ostrom, 1970) one can assume that subjects were differentially committed to either self-evaluations or mood. Possibly subjects who were very high on need for social desirability (Crowne & Marlowe, 1964) experienced a strong demand (Orne, 1962) to use the experimental perspectives normatively and thus were committed to self-evaluations. As a result, they produced the expected judgments even if the outcomes were not represented differently (i.e. there were no effects on their mood).

Other subjects may have shown just the opposite response pattern. If a tendency of consistency in self-evaluations (Deutsch & Solomon, 1959; Swann & Read, 1981) was predominant, subjects may have kept their self-evaluations stable, irrespective of perspective manipulations, but nevertheless changed mood as a result of perspective-dependent changes in stimulus representation. For those subjects who showed changes in self-evaluation but not mood no change in stimulus representation is assumed.

These interpretations would explain why self-evaluations and mood were not intercorrelated in the second experiment. However, alternative explanations are possible.
- Perhaps, because of the neutral response language, no affective judgments (self-evaluations) were measured.
- Self-evaluations as such did not have an effect on mood.

Regarding the first possibility, an evaluatively-laden response language <u>has</u> to be offered for affective judgments to be measured. If this were the case, self-evaluations have been obtained only in our first experiment. Perhaps only cold cognitions, i.e. judgments without self-relevance (Zajonc, 1980), were obtained from the so-called self-evaluation measurement in our second experiment. If so, it would be plausible that judgments did not covary with mood.

Regarding the second possibility, the covariation between self-evaluations and mood in the first experiment was partly due to the effect which judgments had on mood (see the path analyses). Presumably, self-evaluations did not have an effect on mood in the second experiment. One interpretation is that judgments did not have an effect because only cold cognitions were measured with the evaluatively neutral response language (see above). Another is that self-evaluations did not have effects on mood because they were produced under external pressure, namely in the presence of the experimenter who may have communicated a demand to use the experimental perspectives normatively. Such an inter- pretation is consistent with dissonance theory (Festinger, 1957). If a certain behavior, here public self-evaluation, is produced under external pressure, no dissonance results, i.e. mood is not "changed" correspondingly (Wicklund & Brehm, 1968). Alternatively, according to self-perception theory (Bem, 1967, 1972), no internal attitude, i.e. a self-evaluative affect, is "inferred" from behavior under such conditions of external pressure.

Effects of the "life perspective"
In Experiment I, the criterion for an effect of previous judgments on actual ones was clearly met. The skewness of the distribution of standard set ratings was less negative at the second point of measurement.
In both experiments contrast effects resulted from extension of perspectives. Judgments became more negative if the upper anchor was extended. On the other hand, results with respect to the skewness of the distribution are interpreted as indicating that outcome evaluations are assimilated to the modal outcome on a person's life perspective. The more frequent negative evaluations have already occurred, the more negative actual judgments are.

This interpretation is supported by the results of a study from Strack, Schwarz and Gschneidinger (1985). Subjects had to talk about a positive or negative personal event they had experienced in the past. Mood self-ratings ("happiness" and "life satisfaction") were either assimilated or contrasted with the affective quality of the event depending on how a person had talked about it. Contrast effects occurred if the event was mentioned only briefly and if the subject talked about <u>why</u> it had occurred. Assimilation, on the other hand, occurred if the person had talked in a detailed and vivid way about <u>how</u> the event had happened.

Our interpretation is that contrast effects resulted if a 'cold' cognition (Zajonc, 1980) about the event was provoked and assimilation if the cognition was 'hot'.
An internally represented stimulus continuum is extended in the direction of a stimulus a person actually imagines. Accordingly, more positive mood should result if a negative event is remembered and vice versa. On the other hand, assimilation should occur if a 'hot' cognition about an event is activated. To put it into our theoretical terms, the frequency distribution on the life perspective takes effect: self-esteem is used as a correspondence cue since self-esteem corresponds with evaluative events through a value aspect (cf. Upmeyer, 1981, 1982). Applied to achievement situations, 'hot' cognitions about an outcome, i.e. about a <u>self-produced</u> performance result, should lead to assimilation to the global self-esteem of the person. 'Cold' cognitions about performance results, for instance imagination of a <u>possible</u> outcome or about <u>outcomes of other persons</u>, should lead to contrast effects.

Different functions of judgments

Judgments can be conceived of as communicative acts: the internal representation of a certain stimulus is translated onto a given response modality. Our results showed that, under certain conditions, judgments as such have effects on mood, i.e. judgments not only serve a communicative but also an emotion-regulatory function.

Path analyses revealed a direct transmission of perspec- tive- dependent stimulus-perception onto standard set rating, self-evaluations and mood for unthreatened subjects. Judgments in turn did not have any effects on mood. For threatened subjects, however, a parodoxical effect of perspectives on self-evaluations was found. Whereas standard set ratings were more negative in the wide than the narrow perspective condition the opposite held true for self-evaluations. We have interpreted these results as implying a self-protective mechanism preven- ting a negative effect on mood from negative stimulus representation: positively distorted self-evaluations as well as negative standard set ratings had a positive effect on mood. The first result is in line with the assumption that self-serving biases may be emotionally functional (cf. Snyder, Stephan & Rosenfield, 1976; Harvey & Weary, 1981). The second result can be interpreted as empirical evidence that denigrating others may help protect self-esteem (cf. Taylor & Doria, 1981;

Wills, 1981; Lemyre & Smith, 1985; Crocker, Thompson, McGraw & Ingerman, 1987).

Unfortunately, results from the path analytic models in the first experiment could not be replicated in Experiment II because here mood and self-evaluation were not intercorrelated. Since performances were significantly different between experimental groups, the effects of perspectives and performances were confounded in the path model for threatened subjects in Experiment I. Thus, interpretations have to be regarded as preliminary.

Implications for depression research
Our experiments offer only very little empirical support for our theoretical assumptions about the temporal development of stable emotional phenomena. Furthermore, the negative mood states which were induced in our experiments are by no means equivalent with depressive mood. It is conceivable that depressive affects are qualitatively different from negative situational mood. This reservation must be borne in mind, therefore, when considering the following interpretations.

In both our experiments an immediate effect of outcome representation on mood could be shown. These results provide empirical support for outcome-dependent affects

(Weiner, 1985; Metalsky et al., 1987). We have hypothe-sized that some people consistently refer to specific comparison stimuli when judging certain events. If a person consistently takes extremely positive contextual stimuli into account, self-produced performance results are internally represented in a negative fashion. Thus, negative affects may be regarded as conditioned reactions (Leventhal, 1980), given a negative representation of a performance outcome. If own performance results are consistently represented as negative, then negative self-evaluations and affects should occur more often. The finding of an increasing positive skewness in the distribution of standard set ratings may indicate that evaluations become more negative with increasing number of previous negative judgments.

In addition, the causal model for threatened subjects in the first experiment showed an effect of self-evaluations on mood. This demonstrates how self-serving biases can be emotionally functional.

Depressives have been characterized by the absence of self-serving biases (Lewinsohn et al., 1980; Raps et al., 1982; Alloy & Ahrens, 1987; Tennen & Herzberger, 1987). Our results show that negative affects are suppressed by self-serving judgments. This may explain why depressives experience negative affects more frequently. In other studies, it has been shown that depressives differentiate less between the assumptions they make about themselves and other persons (cf. Tabachnik et al., 1983; Pyszczynski, Holt & Greenberg, 1987). Perhaps depressives do not show the self-serving bias of derogating others which our path analyses suggest can have positive effects on mood.

Depressives have been described as having a consistently lowered self-esteem (cf. Pagel & Becker, 1987). Hence, it might even be supposed that depressives would not show the self-protective reactions in response to situationally specific threats to self-esteem which threatened subjects showed in our experiments. Possibly, however, different assumptions have to be made for slightly and severely depressed persons. Ordinarily, the following factors can lead to self-serving reactions (i.e. to positively distorted self-evaluations, and to denigrating others; Tessor & Campbell, 1982):

- the induction of situational depressive mood (Bell, 1978),
- situational threat (cf. Canon, 1964; Skolnick, 1971), and/or
- situationally lowered self-esteem (cf. Frey et al., 1986; Frey & Stahlberg, 1987).

Self-protective reactions, however, would probably not be found in severely depressed people (cf. Ruehlman et al.,

1985). We assume that threat leads to self-protective behavior in nondepressed and slightly depressed people but not in severely depressed persons. For severely depressed people threat should lead to a further intensification of negative mood.

It was found that negative stimulus-representation led to more negative mood if the suppression effect due to positively biased self-evaluations was taken into account.

With respect to the debate in depression research on the question of whether nondepressed or depressed persons show perceptual distortions, the following can be said: Our results favor a view in which the question of whether stimuli are perceived correctly or incorrectly is of secondary importance. If a judgment appears to express a more positive representation of events, this leads to an improvement of mood, regardless of whether this judgment is positively distorted or not. Therefore positively biased self-evaluations may help prevent situational depression (e.g. Klein et al., 1976; Alloy & Ahrens, 1987).

References

Abramson, L.Y. & Alloy, L.B. (1981). Depression, nondepression, and cognitive illusions: A reply to Schwartz. *Journal of Experimental Psychology: General, 110,* 436-447.

Abramson, L.Y., Alloy, L.B. & Metalsky, G.I. (1986). The cognitive diathesis-stress theories of depression: Toward an adequate evaluation of the theories' validities. In L.B. Alloy (Ed.), *Cognitive processes in depression.* New York: Guilford Press.

Abramson, L.Y., Alloy, L.B. & Rosoff, R. (1981). Depression and the generation of complex hypotheses in the judgment of contingency. *Behaviour Research and Therapy, 19,* 35-45.

Abramson, L.Y., Metalsky, G.I. & Alloy, L.B. (1986). The hopelessness theory of depression: Does the research test the theory? In L.Y. Abramson (Ed.), *Social cognition and clinical psychology: A synthesis.* New York: Guilford Press.

Abramson, L.Y., Seligman, M.E.P. & Teasdale, J. (1978). Learned helplessness in humans: Critique and reformulation. *Journal of Abnormal Psychology, 87,* 49-74.

Alloy, L.B. & Abramson, L.Y. (1979). Judgment of contingency in depressed and nondepressed students: Sadder but wiser? *Journal of Experimental Psychology: General, 108,* 441-485.

Alloy, L.B. & Abramson, L.Y. (1982). Learned helplessness, depression, and the illusion of control. *Journal of Personality and Social Psychology, 6,* 1114-1126.

Alloy, L.B., Abramson, L.Y. & Viscusi, D. (1981). Induced mood and the illusion of control. *Journal of Personality and Social Psychology, 41,* 1129-1140.

Alloy, L.B. & Ahrens, A.H. (1987). Depression and pessimism for the future: Biased use of statistically relevant information in predictions for self versus others. *Journal of Personality and Social Psychology, 52,* 366-378.

Asch, S.E. (1946). Forming impressions of personality. *Journal of Abnormal and Social Psychology, 41,* 258-290.

Asch, S.E. (1951). Effects of group pressure upon the modification and distortion of judgment. In Guetzkow, H. (Ed.), *Groups, leadership, and men.* Pittsburg : Carnegie Press.

Atkinson, J.W. (1957). Motivational determinants of risk-taking behavior. *Psychological Review, 64,* 359-372.

Austin, W. (1977). Equity theory and social comparison processes. In J.M. Suls & R.L. Miller (Eds.), *Social comparison processes.* New York: Wiley.

Bandura, A. (1971). *Social learning theory.* Morristown, N.J.: General Learning Press.

Bandura, A. (1974). Behavior theory and the models of man. *American Psychologist, 29,* 859-869.

Bandura, A. (1977). Self-efficacy: Toward a unifying theory of behavioral change. *Psychological Review , 84,* 191-215.

Bandura, A. (1978). The self system in reciprocal determinism. *American Psychologist, 33,* 344-358

Bandura, A. & Cervone, D. (1983). Self-evaluative and self-efficacy mechanisms governing the motivational effects of goal systems. *Journal of Personality and Social Psychology, 45,* 1017-1028.

Bandura, A., Grusec, J.E. & Menlove, F.L. (1967). Observational learning as a function of symbolization and incentive set. *Child Development, 37,* 499-506.

Bandura, A. & Kupers, C. (1964). The transmission of patterns of self-reinforcement through modeling. *Journal of Abnormal and Social Psychology, 69,* 1-9.

Bandura, A. & Whalen, C.K. (1966). The influence of antecedent-reinforcement and divergent modeling cues on patterns of self-reward. *Journal of Personality and Social Psychology, 3,* 373-382.

Barden, R.C., Garber, J., Duncan, S.W. & Masters, J.C. (1981). Cumulative effects of induced affective states in children: Accentuation, inoculation, and remediation. *Journal of Personality and Social Psychology, 40,* 750-760.

Beck, A.T. (1967). *Depression: Clinical, experimental, and theoretical aspects.* New York: Harper and Row.

Beck, A.T. (1976). *Cognitive therapy and the emotional disorders.* New York: International Universities Press.

Bell, P.A.   (1978). Affective state, attraction, and affiliation. *Personality and Social Psychology Bulletin, 4,* 616-619.

Bem, D.J.   (1967). Self-perception: An alternative interpretation of cognitive dissonance phenomena. *Psychological Review, 74,* 183-200.

Bem, D.J.   (1972). Self-perception theory. In L. Berkowitz (Ed.), *Advances in experimental social psychology* (Vol. 6). New York: Academic Press.

Berlyne, D.E.   (1960). *Conflict, arousal, and curiosity.* New York: McGraw-Hill.

Bornewasser, M.   (1985). Verantwortlichkeitsattributionen im Intergruppenkontext am Beispiel deutscher Arbeiter und jugoslawischer Gastarbeiter. *Gruppendynamik. Zeitschrift für angewandte Sozialpsychologie, 16,* 19-33.

Bortz, J.   (1985). *Lehrbuch der Statistik.* Berlin: Springer.

Boski, P.   (1983). Egotism and evaluation in self and other attributions for achievement related outcommes. *European Journal of Social Psychology, 13,* 287-304.

Bower, G.H. (1981). Mood and memory. *American Psychologist, 36,* 129-148.

Brandstädter, J. (1985). Emotion, Kognition, Handlung: Konzeptuelle Beziehungen. In L.H. Eckensberger & E.D. Lantermann (Eds.), *Emotion und Reflexivität.* München: Urban & Schwarzenberg.

Brewer, M.B. & Campbell, D.T. (1976). *Ethnocentrism and intergroup attitudes; East African evidence.* New York: Halstead Press.

Brewin, C.R.   (1985). Depression and causal attributions: What is their relation? *Psychological Bulletin, 98,* 297-309.

Brickman, P. & Bulman, J. (1977). Pleasure and pain in social comparison. In J.M. Suls & R.L. Miller (Eds.), *Social comparison processes.* New York: Wiley.

Brown, D.R.   (1953). Stimulus-similarity and the anchoring of subjective scales. *American Journal of Psychology, 66,* 199-214.

Brown, I. & Inouye, D.K. (1978). Learned helplessness through modeling: The role of perceived similarity in competence. *Journal of Personality and Social Psychology, 36,* 900-908.

Canon, L.K. (1964). Self-confidence and selective exposure to information. In L. Festinger (Ed.), *Conflict, decision, and dissonance.* Stanford, CA: Stanford University Press.

Cochran, S.D. & Hammen, C.L. (1985). Perceptions of stressful life events and depression: A test of attributional models. *Journal of Personality and Social Psychology, 48,* 1562-1571.

Coyne, J.C. (1982). A critique of cognitions as causal entities with particular reference to depression. *Cognitive Therapy and Research, 6,* 3-13.

Coyne, J.C. & Gotlib, I.H. (1983). The role of cognitions in depression: A critical appraisal. *Psychological Bulletin, 94,* 472-505.

Cranach, M. v., Kalbermatten, U., Indermühle, K. & Gugler, B. (1980). *Zielgerichtetes Handeln.* Bern: Huber.

Crocker, J., Thompson, L.L., McGraw, K.M. & Ingerman, C. (1987). Downward comparison, prejudice, and evaluations of others: Effects of self-esteem and threat. *Journal of Personality and Social Psychology, 52,* 907-916.

Crowne, D.P. & Marlowe, D. (1964). *The approval motive.* New York: Wiley.

Deutsch, M. & Solomon, L. (1959). Reactions to evaluations of others as influenced by self-evaluations. *Sociometry, 22,* 93-113.

Dörner, D. (1985). Verhalten, Denken und Emotionen. In L.H. Eckensberger & E.D. Lantermann (Eds.), *Emotion und Reflexivität.* München: Urban & Schwarzenberg.

Dutton, D.G. (1972). Effect of feedback parameters on congruence versus positivity effects in reactions to personal evaluations. *Journal of Personality and Social Psychology, 24,* 266-371.

Edwards, A.L. (1957). *The social desirability variable in personality research.* New York: Dryden.

Eiser, J.R. (1973). Judgement of attitude statements as a function of judges' attitudes and the judgemental dimension. *British Journal of Social and Clinical Psychology, 12,* 231-240.

Eiser, J.R. (1986). *Social Psychology.* Cambridge: University Press.

Eiser, J.R. & Mower White, C.J. (1974). Evaluative consistency and social judgment. *Journal of Personality and Social Psychology, 30,* 349-359.

Eiser, J.R. & Mower White, C.J. (1975). Categorization and congruity in attitudinal judgment. *Journal of Personality and Social Psychology*, *31*, 769-775.

Eiser, J.R. & Osmon, B.F. (1978). Judgmental perspective and the value connotations of response scale labels. *Journal of Personality and Social Psychology*, *36*, 491-497.

Eiser, J.R. & van der Pligt, J. (1982). Accentuation and perspective in attitudinal judgment. *Journal of Personality and Social Psychology*, *42*, 224-238.

Ellis, A. (1962). *Reason and emotion in psychotherapy*. New York: Lyle Stuart.

Erdelyi, M.H. & Appelbaum, G.A. (1973). Cognitive masking: The disruptive effect of an emotional stimulus upon the perception of continguous neutral items. *Bulletin of Psychonomic Society*, *1*, 59-61.

Escalona, S.K. (1940). The effect of success and failure upon the level of aspiration and behavior in manic-depressive psychoses. *University of Iowa: Studies in Child Welfare*, *16*, 199-302.

Festinger, L. (1942). A theoretical interpretation of shifts in level of aspiration. *Psychological Review*, *49*, 235-250.

Festinger, L. (1954). A theory of social comparison processes. *Human Relations*, *7*, 117-140.

Festinger, L. (1957). *A theory of cognitive dissonance*. Stanford, CA:: Stanford University Press.

Filipp, S.H. (1981). Ein allgemeines Modell für die Analyse kritischer Lebensereignisse. In S.H. Filipp (Ed.), *Kritische Lebensereignisse*. München: Urban & Schwarzenberg.

Fishbein, M. & Hunter, R. (1964). Summation versus balance in attitude organisation and change. *Journal of Abnormal and Social Psychology*, *69*, 505-510.

Fitch, G. (1970). Effects of self-esteem, perceived performance, and choice on causal attributions. *Journal of Personality and Social Psychology*, *16*, 311-315.

Frank, J.F. (1935). Individual differences in certain aspects of the level of aspiration. *American Journal of Psychology*, *47*, 119-128.

Frese, M. & Schöfthaler-Rühl, R. (1976). Kognitive Ansätze in der Depressionsforschung. In N. Hoffmann (Ed.), *Depressives Verhalten. Psychologische Modelle der Ätiologie und der Therapie.* Salzburg: Otto Müller Verlag.

Frey, D. & Benning, E. (1983). Das Selbstwertgefühl. In H. Mandl & G. Huber (Eds.), *Emotion und Kognition.* München: Urban & Schwarzenberg.

Frey, D. & Stahlberg, D. (1987). Selection of information after receiving more or less reliable self-threatening information. *Personality and Social Psychology Bulletin, 12,* 434-441.

Frey, D., Stahlberg, D. & Fries, A. (1986). Information seeking of high- and low-anxiety subjects after receiving positive and negative self-relevant feedback. *Journal of Personality, 54,* 694-703.

Friend, R. & Gilbert, J. (1973). Threat and fear of negative evaluation as determinants of locus of social comparison. *Journal of Personality, 41,* 328-340.

Frieze, I.H. & Weiner, B. (1971). Cue utilization and attributional judgments for success and failure. *Journal of Personality, 39,* 591-606.

Gergen, K.J. & Taylor, M.G. (1969). Social expectancy and self-presentation in the status hierarchy. *Journal of Experimental Social Psychology, 5,* 79-92.

Goethals, G.R. & Darley, J.M. (1977). Social comparison theory: An attributional approach. In J.M. Suls & R.L. Miller (Eds.), *Social comparison processes.* New York: Wiley.

Goodhart, D.E. (1986). The effects of positive and negative thinking on performance in an achievement situation. *Journal of Personality and Social Psychology, 51,* 117-124.

Gordon, J.E. (1957). Interpersonal predictions of repressors and sensitizers. *Journal of Personality, 25,* 686-698.

Guilford, J.P. (1954). *Psychometric methods (2nd ed).* New York: McGraw-Hill.

Hakmiller, K.L. (1966). Threat as a determinant of downward comparison. *Journal of Experimental Social Psychology, Supplement 1,* 32-39.

Halisch, F. & Heckhausen, H. (1977). Search for feedback information and effort regulation during task performance. *Journal of Personality and Social Psychology, 35,* 724-733.

Hamilton, D.L. (1969). Responses to cognitive inconsistencies: Personality discrepancy level and response stability. *Journal of Personality and Social Psychology, 11,* 351-362.

Harkins, S.G. & Jackson, J.M. (1985). The role of evaluation in eliminating social loafing. *Personality and Social Psychology Bulletin, 11,* 457-465.

Harvey, D. (1981). Depression and attributional style: Interpretations of important personal events. *Journal of Abnormal Psychology, 90,* 134-142.

Harvey, J.H. & Weary, G. (1981). *Perspectives on attributional processes.* Dubuque: Brown.

Haubensak, G. (1981). Eine Erweiterung der Range-Frequency-Theorie des absoluten Urteils. *Psychologische Beiträge, 23,* 46-64.

Heckhausen, H. (1977). Achievement motivation and its constructs: A cognitive model. *Motivation and Emotion, 1,* 283-329.

Heckhausen, H. (1978). Selbstbewertung nach erwartungswidrigem Leistungsverlauf: Einfluß von Motiv, Kausalattribution und Zielsetzung. *Zeitschrift für Entwicklungspsychologie und Pädagogische Psychologie, 10,* 191-216.

Heckhausen, H. (1980). *Motivation und Handeln.* Heidelberg: Springer.

Helson, H. (1947). Adaptation-level as frame of reference for prediction of psychophysical data. *American Journal of Psychology, 60,* 1-29.

Higgins, E.T. & Lurie, L. (1983). Context, categorization, and recall: The "change-of-standard" effect. *Cognitive Psychology, 15,* 525-547.

Hyman, H.H. (1942). The psychology of status. *Archives of Psychology, Columbia University* (Vol.269).

Ickes, W.J., Wicklund, R.A. & Ferris, C. (1973). Objective self-awareness and self-esteem. *Jorunal of Experimental Social Psychology, 9,* 202-219.

Johnson, H.H. (1966). Some effects of discrepancy level on responses to negative information about one's self. *Sociometry, 29,* 52-66.

Jucknat, M. (1938). Leistung, Anspruchsniveau und Selbstbewußtsein. *Psychologische Forschung, 22*, 89-179.

Kahneman, D. & Miller, D.T. (1986). Norm theory: Comparing reality of its alternatives. *Psychological Review, 83*, 136-153.

Kanfer, F.H. (1970). Self-regulation: Research, issues, and speculations. In C. Neuringer & J.L. Michael (Eds.), *Behavior modification in clinical psychology.* New York: Appleton.

Kanfer, F.H. (1975). Self-management methods. In F.H. Kanfer & A.P. Goldstein (Eds.), *Helping people change.* New York: Pergamon Press.

Kanfer, F.H. & Hagerman, S. (1981). The role of self-regulation. In L.P. Rehm (Ed.), *Behavior therapy for depression: Present status and future directions.* New York: Academic Press.

Karoly, P. & Kanfer, F.H. (1974). Situational and historical determinants of self-reinforcement. *Behavior Therapy, 5*, 381-390.

Katschnig, H. (Ed.), (1980). *Sozialer Streß und psychische Erkrankung.* München: Urban & Schwarzenberg.

Klein, D., Fencil-Morse, E. & Seligman, M.E.P. (1976). Depression, learned helplessness, and the attribution of failure. *Journal of Personality and Social Psychology, 33*, 508-516.

Korman, A.K. (1968). Task success, task popularity and self-esteem as influences on task liking. *Journal of Applied Psychology, 52*, 484-490.

Kuhl, J. (1978). Standard setting and risk preference: An elaboration of the theory of achievement motivation and an empirical test. *Psychological Review, 85*, 239-248.

Kuhl, J. (1983a). *Motivation, Konflikt und Handlungskontrolle.* Berlin: Springer.

Kuhl, J. (1983b). Emotion, Kognition und Motivation: I. Auf dem Wege zu einer systemtheoretischen Betrachtung der Emotionsgenese. *Sprache und Kognition, 2*, 1-27.

Kuhl, J. (1983c). Emotion, Kognition und Motivation: II. Die funktionale Bedeutung der Emotionen für das problem-lösende Denken und für das konkrete Handeln. *Sprache und Kognition, 4*, 228-253.

Kukla, A. (1972). Foundations of an attributional theory of performance. *Psychological Review*, *79*, 454-470.

Lantermann, E.D. (1982). Integration von Kognitionen und Emotionen in Handlungen. In H.W. Hoefert (Ed.), *Interaktionismus*. Göttingen: Hogrefe.

Lantermann, E.D. (1983). Kognitive und emotionale Prozesse beim Handeln. In H. Mandl & G.L. Huber (Eds.), *Emotion und Kognition*. München: Urban & Schwarzenberg.

Latané, B. (1966). Studies in social comparison-Introduction and overview. *Journal of Experimental Social Psychology*, Supplement *1*, 1-5.

Laxer, R. (1964). Self-concept changes of depressive patients in general hospital treatment. *Journal of Consulting Psychology*, *28*, 214-219.

Lemyre, L. & Smith, P.M. (1985). Intergroup discrimination and self-esteem in the minimal intergroup paradigm. *Journal of Personality and Social Psychology*, *49*, 660-670.

Leventhal, H. (1980). Toward a comprehensive theory of emotion. In L. Berkowitz (Ed.), *Advances in experimental social psychology* (Vol. 13). New York: Academic Press.

Leventhal, H. (1984). A perceptual-motor theory of emotion. In L. Berkowitz (Ed.), Advances in experimental and social psychology (Vol. 17). New York: Academic Press.

Lewecki, P. (1983). Self-image bias in person perception. *Journal of Personality and Social Psychology*, *45*, 384-393.

Lewin, K., Dembo, R., Festinger, L. & Sears, P. (1944). Level of aspiration. In J.McV. Hund (Ed.), *Personality and the behavior disorders* (Vol. 1). New York: Ronald Press Co.

Lewinsohn, P.H. (1974). A behavioral approach to depression. In R. Friedman & M. Katz (Eds.), *The psychology of depression: Contemporary theory and research*. Washington, D.C.: Winston-Wiley.

Lewinsohn, P.M., Mischel, W., Chaplain, W. & Barton, R. (1980). Social competence and depression: The role of illusory self-perceptions. *Journal of Abnormal Psychology*, *89*, 203-212.

Lobitz, W.C. & Post, R.D. (1979). Parameters of self-reinforcement and depression. *Journal of Abnormal Psychology, 88*, 33-41.

Loeb, A., Beck, A.T., Diggory, J.C. & Tuthill, R. (1967). Expectancy, level of aspiration, performance, and self-evaluation in depression. *Proceedings of the 75th Annual Convention of the American Psychological Association, 2*, 193-194.

Manis, M. & Paskewitz, J.R. (1984a). Specificity and contrast effects: Judgments of psychopathology. *Journal of Experimental and Social Psychology, 20*, 217-230.

Manis, M. & Paskewitz, J.R. (1984b). Judging psychopathology: Expectation and contrast. *Journal of Experimental and Social Psychology, 20*, 363-381.

Manis, M., Paskewitz, J.R. & Cotler, S. (1986). Stereotypes and social judgment. *Journal of Personality and Social Psychology, 50*, 461-473.

Martin, D.J., Abramson, L.Y. & Alloy, L.B. (1984). Illusion of control for self and others in depressed and nondepressed college students. *Journal of Personality and Social Psychology, 46*, 125-136.

Masters, J.C., Carlson, C.R. & Rahe, D.F. (1985). Children's affective, behavioral, and cognitive responses to social comparison. *Journal of Experimental Social Psychology, 21*, 407-420.

Merton, K.M. & Rossi, A.K. (1949). Contributions to the theory of reference group behavior. In R.K. Merton (Ed.), *Social theory and social structure (rev.ed.)*. New York: The Free Press.

Metalsky, G.I., Abramson, L.Y., Seligman, M.E.P., Semmel, A. & Peterson, C.R. (1982). Attributional styles and life events in the classroom: Vulnerability and invulnerability to depressive mood reactions. *Journal of Personality and Social Psychology, 43*, 612-617.

Metalsky, G.I., Halberstadt, L.J. & Abramson, L.Y. (1987). Vulnerability to depressive mood reactions: Toward a more powerful test of the diathesis-stress and causal mediation components of the reformulated theory of depression. *Journal of Personality and Social Psychology, 52*, 386-393.

Mettee, D.R. & Aronson, E. (1974). Affective reactions to appraisal from others. In T.L. Huston (Ed.), *Foundations of interpersonal attraction.* New York: Academic Press.

Meyer, W.U. (1973). *Leistungsmotiv und Ursachenerklärung von Erfolg und Mißerfolg.* Stuttgart: Klett.

Miller, S.M. (1980). When is a little information a dangerous thing? Coping with stressful life-events by monitoring vs. blunting. In S. Levine & H. Ursin (Eds.), *Coping and health* (pp. 145-169). New York: Plenum Press.

Miller, S.M. (1987). Monitoring and blunting: Validation of a questionnaire to assess styles of information seeking under threat. *Journal of Personality and Social Psychology, 52,* 345-353.

Molleman, E., Pruyn, J. & van Knippenberg, A. (1986). Social comparison processes among cancer patients. *British Journal of Social Psychology, 25,* 1-13.

Morse, S. & Gergen, K.J. (1970). Social comparison, self-consistency, and the concept of self. *Journal of Personality and Social Psychology, 16,* 148-156.

Mummendey, H.D. & Sturm, G. (1978). *Selbstbildänderungen in der Retrospektive: I. Methode und deskriptive Ergebnisse* (Bielefelder Arbeiten zur Sozialpsychologie, 33).

Mummendey, H.D. & Sturm, G. (1980). *Erster Bericht über eine Längsschnittuntersuchung zu kritischen Lebensereignissen und Selbstbildänderungen jüngerer Erwachsener* (Bielefelder Arbeiten zur Sozialpsychologie, 58).

Nadich, M., Gargan, M. & Michael, L. (1975). Denial, anxiety, locus of control, and the discrepancy between aspirations and achievements as components of depression. *Journal of Abnormal Psychology, 84,* 1-9.

Orne, M.T. (1962). On the social psychology of the psychological experiment: With particular reference to demand characteristics and their implications. *American Psychologist, 17,* 776-783.

Ostrom, T.M. (1970). Perspective as a determinant of attitude change. *Journal of Experimental Social Psychology, 6,* 280-292.

Ostrom, T.M. & Upshaw, H.S. (1968). Psychological perspective and attitude change. In A.G. Greenwald; T.C. Brock & T.M. Ostrom (Eds.), *Psychological foundations of attitudes.* New York: Academic Press.

Pagel, M. & Becker, J. (1987). Depressive thinking and depression: Relations with personality and social resources. *Journal of Personality and Social Psychology, 52*, 1043-1052.

Parducci, A. (1963). Range-frequency compromise in judgment. *Psychological Monographs, 77 (2*, whole No. 565).

Parducci, A. (1965). Category judgment: A range-frequency model. *Psychological Review, 72*, 407-418.

Parducci, A. (1984). Value judgments: Toward a relational theory of happiness. In J.R. Eiser (Ed.), *Attitudinal judgment.* New York: Springer.

Parducci, A., Knobel, S. & Thomas, C. (1976). Independent contexts for category ratings: A range-frequency analysis. *Perception and Psychophysics, 20*, 360-366.

Peabody, D. (1967). Trait inferences: Evaluative and descriptive aspects. *Journal of Personality and Social Psychology Monographs, 7* (4, whole No. 644).

Pyszczynski, T., Holt, K. & Greenberg, J. (1987). Depression, self-focused attention, and expectancies for positive and negative future life events for self and others. *Journal of Personality and Social Psychology, 52*, 994-1001.

Raps, C.S., Peterson, C.R., Reinhard, K.E., Abramson, L.Y. & Seligman, M.E.P. (1982). Attributional style among depressed patients. *Journal of Abnormal Psychology, 91*, 102-108.

Ruehlman, L.S., West, S.G. & Pasahow, R.J. (1985). Depression and evaluative schemata. *Journal of Personality, 53*, 46-92.

Sanders, G. (1981). The interactive effect of social comparison and objective information on the decision to see a doctor. *Journal of Applied Social Psychology, 11*, 390-400.

Seta, J. (1982). The impact of comparison processes on coator's task performance. *Journal of Personality and Social Psychology, 42*, 281-291.

Schwarz, N., Hippler, H.J., Deutsch, B. & Strack, F. (1985). Response scales: Effect of category range on reported behavior and comparative judgments. *Public Opinion Quarterly, 49*, 388-395.

Seligman, M.E.P. (1975). *Helplessness. On depression, development, and death.* San Francisco: Freeman.

Shrauger, J.S. & Lund, A.K. (1975). Self-evaluations and reactions to evaluations form others. *Journal of Personality*, *43*, 94-108.

Shrauger, J.S. & Terbovic, M.L. (1976). Self-evaluation and assessments of performance by self and others. *Journal of Consulting and Clinical Psychology*, *44*, 564-572.

Singer, J.E. (1966). Social comparison - Progress and issues. *Journal of Experimental Social Psychology*, Supplement *1*, 103-110.

Skolnick, P. (1971). Reactions to personal evaluations: A failure to replicate. *Journal of Personality and Social Psychology*, *18*, 62-67.

Sledge, W., Boydstun, J. & Rabe, A. (1980). Selfconcept changes related to war captivity. *Archives of General Psychiatry*, *37*, 430-443.

Smedley, J.W. & Bayton, J.A. (1978). Evaluative race-class stereotypes by race and perceived class of subjects. *Journal of Personality and Social Psychology*, *36*, 530-535.

Smolen, R.C. (1978). Expectancies, mood, and performance of depressed and nondepressed psychiatric inpatients on chance and skill tasks. *Journal of Abnormal Psychology*, *87*, 91-101.

Snyder, M.L., Stephan, W.G. & Rosenfield, D. (1976). Egotism and attribution. *Journal of Personality and Social Psychology*, *36*, 435-441.

Stipek, D.J. (1983). A developmental analysis of pride and shame. *Human Development*, *26*, 42-54.

Strack, F., Schwarz, N. & Gschneidinger, E. (1985). Happiness and reminiscing: The role of time perspective, affect, and mode of thinking. *Journal of Personality and Social Psychology*, *49*, 1460-1469.

Stroebe, W. (1977). Self-esteem and interpersonal attraction. In S. Duck (Ed.), *Theory and practice in interpersonal attraction*. London: Academic Press.

Swann, W.B. & Read, S.J. (1981). Self-verification processes: How we strain our self-conceptions. *Journal of Experimental Social Psychology*, *17*, 351-372.

Tabachnik, N., Crocker, J. & Alloy, L. (1983). Depression, social comparison, and the false-consensus effect. *Journal of Personality and Social Psychology*, *45*, 688-699.

Taylor, D.M. & Doria, J.R. (1981). Self-serving and group serving bias in attribution. *Journal of Social Psychology, 113,* 201-211.

Taylor, S.E. & Brown, J. (1986). *Illusion and well-being: Some social psychological contributions to a theory of mental health.* (Manuscript submitted for publication).

Taylor, S.E., Wood, J.V. & Lichtman, R.R. (1983). It could be worse: Selective evaluation as a response to victimization. *Journal of Social Issues, 39,* 19-40.

Tennen, H. & Herzberger, S. (1987). Depression, self-esteem, and the absence of self-protective attributional biases. *Journal of Personality and Social Psychology, 52,* 72-80.

Tesser, A. (1984). Self-evaluation maintenance processes: Implications for relationships and for development. In J.C. Masters & K. Yarkin-Levin (Eds.), *Boundary areas in social and developmental psychology.* London: Academic Press.

Tesser, A. & Campbell (1980). Self-definition: The impact of the relative performance and similarity of others. *Social Psychology Quarterly, 43,* 341-347.

Tesser, A. & Campbell, J. (1982). Self-evaluation maintenance and the perception of friends and strangers. *Journal of Personality, 50,* 261-279.

Thornton, D.A. & Arrowood, A.J. (1966). Self-evaluation, self-enhancement, and the locus of social comparison. *Journal of Experimental Social Psychology,* Supplement *1,* 40-48.

Toda, M., Shinotsuka, H., McClintock, C.G. & Stech, F.J. (1978). Development of competitive behavior as a function of culture, age, and social comparison. *Journal of Personality and Social Psychology, 36,* 825-829.

Upmeyer, A. (1976). Ethnische Identifikation. *Zeitschrift für Sozialpsychologie, 7,* 143-153.

Upmeyer, A. (1981). Perceptual and judgmental processes in social contexts. In L. Berkowitz (Ed.), *Advances in experimental social psychology* (Vol. 14). New York: Academic Press.

Upmeyer, A. (1982). Attitudes and social behavior. In J.P. Codol & J.P. Leyens (Eds.), *Cognitive analysis of social behavior.* Den Haag: Nijhoff-Martinus.

Upshaw, H.S. (1962). Own attitude as an anchor in equal-appearing intervals. *Journal of Abnormal and Social Psychology, 64,* 85-96.

Upshaw, H.S. (1969a). The personal reference scale: An approach to social judgment. In L. Berkowitz (Ed.), *Advances in experimental social psychology* (Vol. 4). New York: Academic Press.

Upshaw, H.S. (1969b). Stimulus range and judgmental unit. *Journal of Experimental Social Psychology, 5,* 1-11.

Upshaw, H.S. (1978). Social influence on attitudes and on anchoring of congeneric attitude scales. *Journal of Experimental Social Psychology, 14,* 327-339.

Upshaw, H.S. & Ostrom, T.M. (1984). Psychological perspective in attitude research. In J.R. Eiser (Ed.), *Attitudinal judgment.* New York: Springer.

Vázquez, C. (1987). Judgment of contingency: Cognitive biases in despressed and nondepressed subjects. *Journal of Personality and Social Psychology, 52,* 419-431.

Volkmann, J. (1951). Scales of judgment and their implications for social psychology. In J.H. Rohrer & M. Sherif (Eds.), *Social psychology at the crossroads.* New York: Harper & Row.

Weiner, B. (1974). *Achievement motivation and attribution theory.* Morristown, N.J.: General Learning Press.

Weiner, B. (1980). *Human motivation.* New York: Holt, Rinehart and Winston.

Weiner, B. (1985). An attributional theory of achievement motivation and emotion. *Psychological Review, 92,* 548-573.

Weiner, B. & Handel, S. (1985). Anticipated emotional consequences of causal communications and reported communication strategy. *Developmental Psychology, 21,* 102-107.

Weiner, B. & Kukla, A. (1970). An attributional analysis of achievement motivation. *Journal of Personality and Social Psychology, 15,* 1-20.

Wicklund, R.A. & Brehm, J.W. (1968). Attitude change as a function of felt competence and threat to attitudinal freedom. *Journal of Experimental Social Psychology, 4,* 64-75.

Wills, T.A. (1981). Downward comparison principles in social psychology. *Psychological Bulletin, 90,* 245-271.

Wilson, S.R. & Benner, L.A. (1971). The effects of self-esteem and situation upon comparison choices during ability evaluation. *Sociometry, 34,* 381-397.

Wollert, R., Heinrich, L., Wood, D. & Werner, W. (1983). Causal attributions, sanctions, and normal mood variations. *Journal of Personality and Social Psychology, 45,* 1029-1044.

Wood, J., Taylor, S. & Lichtman, R. (1985). Social comparison in adjustment to breast cancer. *Journal of Personality and Social Psychology, 49,* 1169-1183.

Wyer, R.S. & Frey, D. (1983). The effects of feedback about self and others on the recall and judgments of feedback-relevant information. *Journal of Experimental Social Psychology, 19,* 540-559.

Zajonc, R.B. (1980). Feeling and thinking. Preferences need no inferences. *American Psychologist, 35,* 151-175.

Zavalloni, M. & Cook, S.W. (1965). Influence of judges' attitudes on ratings of favorableness of statements about a social group. *Journal of Personality and Social Psychology, 1,* 43-54.

Zerssen, D. (1976). *Klinische Selbstbeurteilungs-Skalen (KSb-S) aus dem Münchener Psychiatrischen Informations-System (PSYCHIS München). Die Befindlichkeitsskala - Parallelformen Bf-S und Bf-S'.* Weinheim: Beltz Test Gesellschaft mbH.